# ICU Management and Protocols

*Edited by Nissar Shaikh and Theodoros Aslanidis*

Published in London, United Kingdom

ICU Management and Protocols
http://dx.doi.org/10.5772/intechopen.98095
Edited by Nissar Shaikh and Theodoros Aslanidis

Contributors
Artem A. Aleksandrovich Ivkin, Evgeny V. Grigoryev, Naadiyah Laher, Ballah Abubakar, Jacob Dunga, Yusuf B. Jibrin, Buma Bordiya, Ibrahim Maigari, Hassan Maina, Jean Maxime Côté, Dominic Godbout, Philippe Lachance, Suzanne Crowe, Maeve McAllister, Dhruv Talwar, Sunil Kumar, Deepak Talwar, Rungrote Natesirinilkul



First published in London, United Kingdom, 2022 by IntechOpen
IntechOpen is the global imprint of INTECHOPEN LIMITED, registered in England and Wales, registration number: 11086078, 5 Princes Gate Court, London, SW7 2QJ, United Kingdom

British Library Cataloguing-in-Publication Data
A catalogue record for this book is available from the British Library

Additional hard and PDF copies can be obtained from orders@intechopen.com

ICU Management and Protocols
Edited by Nissar Shaikh and Theodoros Aslanidis
p. cm.
Print ISBN 978-1-80355-936-0
Online ISBN 978-1-80355-937-7
eBook (PDF) ISBN 978-1-80355-938-4

# Meet the editors

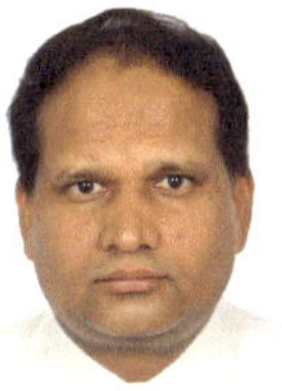

Dr. Nissar Shaikh, MD, EDIC, DID, FCCM, is a senior intensive care consultant and surgical intensive care fellowship director at Hamad Medical Corporation, Qatar. He is an assistant professor at Weill Cornell Medicine-Qatar and an associate professor at the College of Medicine, Qatar University. Dr. Nissar has made numerous oral and poster presentations at national and international conferences. He has 150 peer-reviewed publications in critical and acute care to his credit as well as 3 books and 30 book chapters. He has won three prestigious awards for distinguished services from Hamad Medical Corporation.

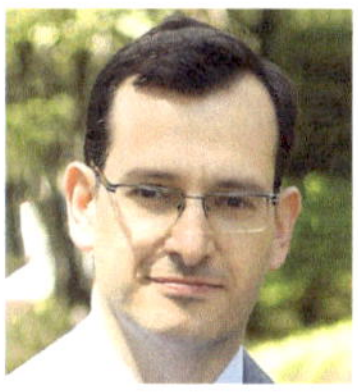

Theodoros Aslanidis received his Doctor of Medicine degree from Plovdiv Medical University, Bulgaria, and his Ph.D. from Aristotle University, Thessaloniki, Greece. After serving as a medical doctor in the Hellenic Armed Forces and as a rural physician in Outhealth Centre, Iraklia and Serres General Hospital, Greece, he completed specialist anesthesiology training at Ippokrateio General Hospital, Thessaloniki, critical care sub-specialty training at AHEPA University Hospital, and a Prehospital Emergency Medicine postgraduate program at the Hellenic National Centre for Emergency Care. He served as an EMS physician and emergency communication center medic before moving to his current post as consultant-researcher in the Intensive Care Unit at St. Paul General Hospital, Thessaloniki. He is also a senior lecturer at the College of Offshore and Remote Medicine, Pretty Bay, Malta.

# Contents

# Preface

*ICU Management and Protocols* describes the management of acute and critically ill patients. It discusses important topics in intensive care practices for both adult and pediatric patients. Chapters address professionalism and teamwork in the intensive care setup, various modalities of renal replacement therapy in critically ill patients, the management of postoperative delirium and coagulopathies in pediatric patients, and resuscitation of trauma and mass casualty patients during the COVID-19 pandemic.

This book is a useful resource for intensive care physicians, emergency physicians, acute care and general surgeons, EMS staff, and acute and critical care nurses.

We are thankful to Ms. Ana Cink for her continuous help at all stages of the publication process. I am indebted and thankful to Dr. Firdous for her support and encouragement during the editing process. I am also grateful for the patience and cooperation of my daughters Dr. Amara and Dr. Jaza. Finally, I wish to acknowledge the participating authors for their valuable contributions.

**Dr. Nissar Shaikh**
Hamad Medical Corporation,
Doha, Qatar

**Theodoros Aslanidis**
Saint Paul General Hospital of Thessaloniki,
Thessaloniki, Greece

Chapter 1

# Professionalism, Teamwork and Regulation in the Intensive Care Unit

*Suzanne Crowe and Maeve McAllister*


## Abstract

In this chapter, we discuss the concepts of professionalism in relation to intensive care medicine. The intensive care management of patients represents the sharp edge of every speciality and the potential for miscommunication, conflict, psychological overload and burnout is large. The presence of a culture of trust between patients and staff, and between staff members is a major factor in patient outcome, staff recruitment, staff retention and motivation. As critical care morbidity and mortality rates improve, patient and staff expectations of an acceptable short-term and long-term outcome increase. To reach these expectations, healthcare professionals need to operate in high performing teams, with defined standards and objectives. We focus on key aspects of good professional behaviour, high-performance healthcare teams and the regulatory aspects of care in the high technology, critical care environment.


**Keywords:** critical care, intensive care, professionalism, teamwork, regulation

## 1. Introduction

Critical care medicine offers many challenges for staff and patients. When admitted to the Intensive Care Unit (ICU) patients are critically ill and require life-saving intervention with the aim of disease treatment and maximising organ support and recovery. If the patient survives, there may be a prolonged period of rehabilitation. This level of medical intervention is usually coordinated by a specialist in critical care medicine and delivered by a multidisciplinary team of health professionals.

The range of disciplines that now contribute to the outcome of the patient has grown and includes clinical psychology, speech and language therapy, bioengineering and clinical pharmacy. As care has become more complex, the need for experienced professionals has increased, with a worldwide shortage of intensive care staff. Recruitment, training and retention of valuable ICU staff are important. Understanding what makes team members satisfied with their job is vital in keeping good staff, reducing disruptive staff turnover and improved continuity of high-quality care to patients. Emphasis on a healthy professional culture within the ICU can be helpful in encouraging personal and professional development, and positive interactions between staff and patients.

## 2. Professionalism

The term professionalism describes the attributes of a skilled competent practitioner. These qualities reassure the patient and their family that they can trust healthcare staff to do their best for them, be honest in their interactions and speak up when needed. Professionalism also encompasses an acceptance that a clinician participates in ongoing training and education, reflective practice, audit and assessment. Within its scope is a code of conduct which always prioritises the dignity and safety of the patient.

## 3. Teamwork

As we have moved from parallel practice to the concept of integrative multidisciplinary care, the intensive care team has evolved to include many physicians and healthcare professionals who share the common goal of delivering high quality, coordinated patient-centred care. Team members are highly skilled professionals who contribute from their diverse knowledge and experiences to improve patient care.

The structure of the team can vary depending on the needs of the patient and the availability of staff. During a typical admission to the intensive care unit (ICU) a patient can expect to receive care from the following team members; ICU doctor, ICU nurse, medical/surgical doctor, physiotherapist, dietician, occupational therapist, speech and language therapist, pharmacist, psychologist and social worker. The delivery of patient care is the result of a highly coordinated effort from each of these professionals. Many critical care units will be in teaching hospitals, so there will be students and trainees in each discipline present and participating in the team. With healthcare staff delivering care over 24-hour periods, there is a handover of patient information across shifts. This means relatively large numbers of trained staff are required to maintain safe care. To operate a large team in a cohesive fashion takes attention and a proactive approach to resolving differences in opinion. Excellent communication assists greatly in keeping a team together, with the common aim of giving good patient care.

### 3.1 High performance teams in the intensive care unit

There is an emerging body of research, which suggests that high-performance teams lead to improved outcomes in healthcare. Initially coined in the 1950s and adopted as a concept within organisation development, a high-performance team consist of a group of skilled individuals with a shared goal. The analogy has been drawn from Formula 1 motor racing and nuclear energy production. All high-performance teams are under pressure to deliver consistently high-quality results in a climate of significant risk. Through open communication, role expectations and group operating procedures, the high-performance team collaborate to produce reliable superior results.

Considering the wide variety of expertise amongst professionals involved in delivering critical care, the concept of a high-performance team seems appropriate to adopt. In this section, we discuss the essential components of high-performance teamwork and the potential barriers faced in the busy intensive care environment.

### *3.1.1 Fundamental elements of high-performance teamwork in the intensive care unit*

#### *3.1.1.1 Common goals*

The ICU team must agree upon short- and long-term goals of care for each patient. These goals are individualised and reflect the priorities of the patient and their family. All team members, including the family, should be involved in the initial setting of goals of care. Ideally, these goals should be written down and be easily accessible to all team members. There should be regular and routine evaluation of progress and all team members must agree on amendment of processes if goals are not sufficiently reached.

#### *3.1.1.2 Clear roles and responsibilities*

Each member of the ICU team must have individual, discipline-specific roles, and responsibilities. It is important that team members are aware of each other's functions, so each has a clear understanding of both individual and team obligations. Labour should be divided according to the expertise available to enhance team efficiency in realising common goals. Holding information in separate silos across the ICU team may cause difficulties in communication, especially out of usual working hours. For this reason, it is preferable if clinical records are contributed to and maintained centrally. This is easy to achieve when an electronic record is used.

#### *3.1.1.3 Accountability*

High-performance teams must demonstrate individual and shared accountability. Individual accountability is dependent upon the personal values of each team member. It may be encouraged by setting personal goals for team members and regular feedback to the individual. Shared accountability can be achieved by agreeing upon group-wide operating rules and standards. Regular review and reinforcement of standards will encourage mutual accountability amongst the team. Open discussion of risk, adverse events and error is a key element in producing accountability: if critical care staff feel that they work in a climate of compassionate understanding of adverse events, they are more likely to be comfortable managing their personal responsibility for patient care.

#### *3.1.1.4 Leadership*

Effective teams require a team leader who is responsible for overseeing group performance. The team leader should ensure provision of a cohesive and supportive team environment. Although traditionally the physician would be the team lead in ICU, the lead in any given scenario may be determined by the needs and experience of the team at that time, rather than in a hierarchical manner. Shared decision making is fundamental to a high-performance team. The team leader should abolish the top-down leadership style and encourage every team member to have a voice, regardless of their position. The value of this approach becomes clear as the team develops and leads to richer interaction. When a critical incident occurs that requires flat lines of communication and prompt action, prior investment of time and effort in professionalism development across the team delivers excellent results in terms of patient care and how team members feel after the event. If there is a poor outcome, follow up between the team leader and team members is important to support staff and extract learnings that can be shared with the aim of improving care.

*3.1.1.5 Continual enhancement of skills*

Team members must commit to continual enhancement of their individual skills. This may involve participation in courses or further academic endeavours. The high performing team will encourage each member to enhance their skills and provide adequate time and support for such activities. Team-based education and simulation sessions can facilitate learning in an environment with considerable risk of serious adverse events [1–3]. Interdisciplinary education may also improve team bonding and communication [4].

*3.1.1.6 Wellbeing*

Individual and team wellbeing must be acknowledged by the institution. High personal and collective morale may enhance job satisfaction. This can in turn improve collaborative processes, productivity, and staff retention.

*3.1.1.7 Psychological safety*

To function at a high level, trust between team members is imperative. Psychological safety is the belief that one will not be punished or humiliated for making suggestions or admitting to error. This encourages transparency amongst team members. A no-blame culture is fostered where active participation and critical thinking can flourish, allowing the team to discuss and learn from their mistakes [5]. This collaborative approach will address deficits in the team's processes to improve the safety of patient care. Maintaining the dignity of a patient in the critical care unit is central to good care. Placing an emphasis on the dignity of staff is important to staff psychological safety and retention. Each unit needs to have active measures in place to tackle bullying. Bullying is extremely damaging and contributes to high staff turnover, which impacts patient care. Focus on upstream measures is most effective—creating a positive culture of support for each other at a fundamental human level exposes those who begin to engage in bullying as being out of step with the 'norm' for this unit. This approach includes coaching and mentoring through addressing errors, and remediation to keep staff working safely. All team members should be encouraged to care for themselves emotionally and physically, with institutional promotion of self-care, good mental health and collegial conduct.

*3.1.1.8 Conflict management*

Open communication is essential for high-performing teams. A diverse multidisciplinary team may have conflicting individual ideas or priorities at times. Team members must feel comfortable and supported to communicate their concerns about team processes and direction of patient care. The team must have consistent channels for communication, ideally with regularly scheduled meetings. Conflicting ideas must be identified and discussed early. It is important for the team leader to embrace but depersonalise diverse views. They will manage relationships amongst the team members and address any obstacles that may hinder group performance. Professionalism supports should be funded and made available including specific training courses, facilitated debriefing, mentoring and referral to counselling. These measures may be co-facilitated by the human resources department in the hospital, as there may be overlap with employment issues.

#### *3.1.1.9 Outcome measurement*

Any high-performance team should have a measurement system in place to determine their success. This allows for timely and reliable feedback to the team regarding their successes and failures. Local metrics foster an environment of continual improvement and learning. Most intensive care units collect a vast amount of data on patient admissions, and this contributes to audits. Intensive care units may collaborate and combine their audit information to produce more robust targets and standards e.g., Paediatric Intensive Care Audit Network (PicaNet) in the United Kingdom and Ireland. This means that measurable patient care processes can be audited against the group's agreed standards and amendments made to local processes based upon results. An example of this is the assessment of an unplanned extubation event. Using data from a number of ICUs and from a number of years, it is possible to produce a standardised rate and compare individual units performance each year against this rate. Ideally, outcomes would be validated and internationally recognised to allow the team to compare themselves with similar units in other jurisdictions [6]. Patient's outcomes can be tracked over time and communicated back to the team. Satisfaction of patients, their families and team members can also be measured and followed over time. Staff resigning from work should be offered a confidential interview to ascertain information which might assist in improving team-working and patient care.

#### *3.1.1.10 Appraisal of team members*

Feedback to individuals and the team reinforces positive behaviours and allows for continual development of the team. It also provides an opportunity for deficits to be identified and remediated. A 360-evaluation process may be utilised whereby many colleagues, regardless of discipline or seniority, will provide evaluation for a team member [7]. Interpersonal skills and professionalism are the core emphasis of this approach.

#### *3.1.1.11 Research*

ICU team members must keep up to date with the latest emerging evidence in their respective fields. Critical care medicine is a technology-dependent speciality which is rapidly evolving. Specific assessment of new techniques, medications and equipment should be incorporated into a local coordinated research agenda. This is necessary to achieve continuously improving, team-based healthcare. Team members must be provided with sufficient time and resources to engage in relevant research, and feedback their results into clinical practice.

#### *3.1.1.12 The patient and family as team members*

Vital to a high-performing ICU team is the inclusion of the patient and their family as integral members of the team. This concept of shared decision-making is gradually replacing a more paternalistic style of directing care [8]. It is important to involve the family in clinical decision making and to allocate sufficient time to meet with them. The patient's needs and expectations are the driving force for the team's efforts, and some neonatal and paediatric intensive care units now facilitate unrestricted family visiting and limited participation in medical rounds.

### *3.1.2 Barriers to high-performance teamwork in the intensive care unit*

#### *3.1.2.1 The changing team*

As staff change from day to night shift and junior doctors rotate through training posts, the multidisciplinary ICU team is continually changing. Although some team members will be a constant presence, the changing nature of the team can threaten its performance [9]. It may be difficult for new team members to join a well-established and experienced team and it takes time and effort for team members to build a trusting relationship with each other. The rotation of care providers may also influence the continuity of care delivered to the patient. This highlights the importance of having established written goals for patient care.

#### *3.1.2.2 Interpersonal relationships*

With the amalgamation of many personalities and healthcare specialities, it is inevitable that conflict may occur within the ICU team. Tension may arise due to the existence of differing priorities or perspectives of team members [10]. Occasionally, the priorities of the team may not align with those of the patient or family. The relationship between team members and the patient and family is important in the overall delivery of care, job satisfaction and incidence of compassion fatigue. Tensions can be exacerbated by inefficient or infrequent communication between team members—this contributes to disharmony in the patient's bedspace, especially if conflicting pieces of information and opinions are being passed onto the patient and their family. Although reaching an agreement between all team members is challenging, it can be facilitated with early and open communication. Senior team members must oversee conflict resolution with maturity and compassion [11, 12].

#### *3.1.2.3 Psychological stress*

The ICU can be a demanding work environment which poses several challenges to team members. Caring for a critically unwell child and their family can be distressing. Team members are often faced with stressful resuscitations, emergencies, and death. Ethical dilemmas are often encountered and can have a psychological impact on the staff involved. A supportive environment is essential to allow staff members to manage these stressors and continue to function as a high-performing team. Debriefing should be used after critical incidents and staff should have access to a counselling service.

#### *3.1.2.4 Resource limitations*

Whilst dependent largely upon the collaborative efforts of individual team members, a high-performance healthcare team does require organisational support to function maximally. Adequate resources must be in place to support the work of the team. Health informatics and technological resources should facilitate seamless communication between team members. Financial support should be in place to allow for education and research. Appropriate facilities should be provided for team meetings, education sessions and simulation. Medical equipment should meet minimum standards to deliver care. Team members should be provided with adequate time for completion of clinical duties, continual professional development, and rest.

### 3.2 Regulatory aspects of medical care in the intensive care unit

Regulation of medical practice in any speciality should focus on 'right touch'. This is a balance between onerous rules which may lead to defensive practice and light-touch regulation which may not be sufficient to guide good practice. Moving the emphasis of regulation upstream, to the issues which can positively impact a physician's professionalism will potentially reduce the number and significance of breaches of conduct and competence. Many regulatory bodies around the world now use this 'right touch' approach to medical regulation. There has been a move away from self-regulation in many jurisdictions, with the establishment of statutory bodies with a non-medical majority. This is a deliberate action to give reassurance to patients that public protection is the key remit of regulation.

In consultation with the public and the profession, high standards of education and practice are developed. These high standards of medical undergraduate and postgraduate education, postgraduate and speciality training, medical ethics and communication are then applied to educational institutions and individual doctors. Following assessment, recommendations for domains of improvement are made by the regulatory authority and followed up in a cycle of appropriate, targeted regulation. Tailored guides to specific areas of medical practice may be produced by a medical regulator to inform doctors and the public of the standards expected e.g., Telemedicine. A regulator will usually maintain a register of doctors who are qualified in that profession. That register is open to the public for inspection and assurance.

The Intensive Care Unit is a key part of a hospital environment. Intensive or critical care medicine has expanded over the last 2 decades to include premature neonates (Neonatology), infants and children (Paediatric Intensive Care) and adults (Adult ICU). Most ICUs will provide education and training to medical practitioners as part of structured training programs. The curriculum and formal assessment of the training program are decided by the certifying professional body e.g., European Society of Intensive Care Medicine (ESICM). A hospital and its medical staff will have a relationship with a medical regulatory body to ensure that there is protection of the public interest in its interactions with doctors employed within the hospital. All doctors must demonstrate their licence or registration with their regulatory body as part of their terms of employment. This provides the public with confidence that their doctor has the necessary medical qualifications to provide medical services.

#### *3.2.1 Education and training*

Regulation extends into education and training with the setting of standards and the periodic evaluation of these standards by the regulatory body. In the ICU, all doctors are expected to meet a basic standard of medical practice and conduct, in addition to demonstrating ongoing learning. There may be overlap with individual training programs and a sharing of compliance data. Accreditation of training bodies by the regulator may be a feature of some healthcare systems, but the principles are the same. A doctor may be asked to demonstrate fitness to practice through a process of investigation if there is a significant complaint made against the doctor. Management of a complaint against a professional is outlined below in Section 2.7.

### 3.2.2 Continued professional development

Each doctor working in the critical care environment has a professional and ethical obligation to keep up to date with clinical developments. Each year specific training courses may be mandated e.g., resuscitation procedures and algorithms. Professional competencies in communication are important in the ICU where giving patients and families bad news is a vital part of the senior medical role. Miscommunication is a common area of complaint where families have a grievance around how important information was imparted by a doctor. There are simulation modules and training drills in communication skills available.

### 3.2.3 Supervision and revalidation

All doctors in training programs must be supervised by a doctor senior in experience. Supervision is a skilled intervention, providing oversight of clinical activity, guidance and the capacity for feedback and debriefing. Doctors of all training levels and ability should have access to a supervisor. As critical care medicine is an acute speciality where patients' clinical status can deteriorate rapidly, supervision should be accessible 24/7. Doctors returning to clinical practice in the ICU following a significant period of absence should be asked to work within a structured program of revalidation to ensure that the doctor is ready to return to full practice and deliver safe patient care. This revalidation program may be sourced from within larger intensive care units, or from the doctor's professional body.

### 3.2.4 Mentoring

A mentor can have the capacity to listen and support a colleague and is a formal professionalism arrangement. Informal collegial behaviour is important but not guaranteed, so developing a mentoring relationship over time can assist a physician who needs career advice or advice on managing conflict or clinically challenging situations. Training programs frequently assign a formal mentor to new entrants, however comfortable mentoring relationships often grow organically.

### 3.2.5 Duty of Candour

In some countries or states, doctors have a legal obligation to disclose details of adverse clinical events to patients and their families. In most areas of clinical practice, there is an ethical duty on the physician to openly discuss significant events or information which could impact patient care. Doctors in the ICU are supported in disclosing information with the support of senior hospital management. Meetings with patients where such matters are disclosed should be documented clearly in the patient's medical record. The patient should be offered psychological support and follow up after any adverse event.

### 3.2.6 Raising concerns

All doctors have an ethical duty to document and voice concerns, with regard to clinical resources, patient care and community care of the patient. Safeguarding of patients involves a legal mandate in many countries to formally report a concern that a vulnerable patient is being subjected to abuse. Patients in ICU are vulnerable because of their critical illness and sedation levels which will generally compromise their capacity to advocate for themselves. If a doctor feels that they do not have access to the resources to safely care for their patients, they should clearly articulate this deficit in writing to senior management within their institution. Risk to patient's care is an important issue in the critical care environment. There are many publications cataloguing incidences of preventable patient harm, and it is a significant cost to the healthcare system in terms of litigation.

#### *3.2.7 Managing a complaint*

Patients in ICU and their families may make a complaint about the care that they have received, or their outcome. Sometimes disagreements about direction of care or interventions can occur and it is wise to invest time into resolving potential disputes as soon as they arise. There are a small number of situations that will result in a formal complaint to hospital management even in the context of good quality patient care. Learning the tools to respond compassionately to a complaint, answer questions and give further information is vital to the doctor working in the high-pressure ICU environment. Having access to specific institutional supports is useful if they exist—some hospitals will have a Patient Support Unit or Complaints Department that can assist in open communication with patients and their families. When a complaint is received it is crucial to take adequate time to review the patient's medical information and clinical course in ICU before responding. A calm response with an expression of empathy is essential. If possible, offer to meet the complainant to discuss the issue to their satisfaction. Both parties should have an accompanying support person, and the meeting should be documented. Open disclosure of facts is expected by complainants and their right to information must be respected. If there has been a poor outcome, this should be acknowledged, and further support offered.

#### *3.2.8 Preparation of reports*

Patients who have been in the ICU occasionally warrant a report on their course in ICU. This may be requested by insurance companies, legal representatives or the Coroner. Reports should be prepared by the senior critical care physician involved in the admission of the patient to the ICU. Adequate time should be assigned to the task, with full access to clinical records. It is wise for the report to confine itself to the facts of the case and refrain from opinion unless specifically asked for. Preparation of a report may elicit a request to attend a court hearing to present the information, and this should be allowed as part of the duties of a senior doctor working in ICU.

## 4. Conclusions

1. Professionalism and effective teamworking are key features of high-quality critical care medicine and contribute to improved patient care.

2. Understanding the regulation of educational and training standards in the intensive care unit is important to ensure that medical care is delivered in an environment which is routinely inspected and accredited.

## Acknowledgements

No external funds were sought or obtained for the preparation of this manuscript.

## Conflict of interest

The authors declare no conflict of interest.

## Author details

Suzanne Crowe* and Maeve McAllister
Senior Fellow in Pediatric Anesthesiology, Children's Health, Dublin, Ireland

*Address all correspondence to: suzanne.crowe@olchc.ie

## References

[1] Salas E, Paige JT, Rosen MA. Creating new realities in healthcare: The status of simulation-based training as a patient safety improvement strategy. BMJ Quality and Safety. 2013;**22**(6):449-452

[2] Cook DA, Hatala R, Brydges R, Zendejas B, Szostek JH, Wang AT, et al. Technology-enhanced simulation for health professions education: A systematic review and meta-analysis. Journal of the American Medical Association. 2011;**306**(9):978-988

[3] Stocker M, Allen M, Pool N, De Costa K, Combes J, West N, et al. Impact of an embedded simulation team training programme in a paediatric intensive care unit: A prospective, single-centre, longitudinal study. Intensive Care Medicine. 2012;**38**(1):99-104

[4] Hammick M, Freeth D, Koppel I, Reeves S, Barr H. A best evidence systematic review of interprofessional education: BEME Guide no. 9. Medical Teacher. 2007;**29**(8):735-751

[5] Edmondson AC. Learning from failure in health care: Frequent opportunities, pervasive barriers. Quality & Safety in Health Care. 2004;**13**(Suppl. 2):3-9

[6] Verburg IWM, de Jonge E, Peek N, de Keizer NF. The association between outcome-based quality indicators for intensive care units. PLoS One. 2018;**13**(6):e0198522

[7] Tumerman M, Carlson LM. Increasing medical team cohesion and leadership behaviors using a 360-degree evaluation process. WMJ. 2012;**111**(1):33-37

[8] Hawryluck LA, Espin SL, Garwood KC, Evans CA, Lingard LA. Pulling together and pushing apart: Tides of tension in the ICU team. Academic Medicine. 2002;**77**(10 Suppl):S73-S76

[9] Weller JM, Torrie J, Boyd M, Frengley R, Garden A, Ng WL, et al. Improving team information sharing with a structured call-out in anaesthetic emergencies: A randomized controlled trial. British Journal of Anaesthesia. 2014;**112**(6):1042-1049

[10] Kayser JB, Kaplan LJ. Conflict Management in the ICU. Critical Care Medicine. 2020;**48**(9):1349-1357

[11] Marinelli AM. Can regulation improve safety in critical care? Critical Care Clinics. 2005;**21**(1):149-162

[12] Wheeler R. Candour for surgeons: The absence of spin. Annals of the Royal College of Surgeons of England. 2014;**96**(6):420-422

Chapter 2

# Non-Invasive Ventilation in Acute Hypoxemic Respiratory Failure

*Dhruv Talwar, Sunil Kumar and Deepak Talwar*


## Abstract

Non-invasive Ventilation (NIV) has emerged as an useful aid for management of pulmonary diseases specifically in cases of respiratory failure. NIV provides respiratory support without the need of an endotracheal tube, helping in avoiding the complications associated with intubation such as tracheal trauma, infection, bleeding, injury to the lung tissues and aspiration. NIV has turned out to provide substantial benefit in the management of chronic obstructive pulmonary disease, acute respiratory distress syndrome, cardiogenic pulmonary edema and in cases of neuromuscular disorders. It has now become an integral tool in the management of respiratory failure, both at home as well as hospital settings including critical care units. All patients of respiratory failure irrespective of causes likeAcute exacerbations of COPD, Acute pulmonary edema, Exacerbations of cystic fibrosis, asthma, or restrictive lung disease and Pneumonia admitted in intensive care unit/high dependent units are suitable for NIV. Noninvasive ventilation is standard of care in chronic respiratory failure and has replaced invasive ventilation in such settings. Its flexibility in use and ease of administration allows it to be acceptable by patients as well as caregivers.


**Keywords:** non-invasive ventilation, acute hypoxic respiratory failure, Bilevel positive airway pressure, portable ventilator, negative pressure ventilation

## 1. Introduction

Brief History: Till mid-20th century Non-invasive Ventilation (NIV) was the mainstay of mechanical ventilatory assistance and it was delivered by negative pressure devices such as the "iron lung" that was used predominantly for poliomyelitis patients with respiratory paralysis. Ironically when its demand and supply suffered during the polio epidemic in Denmark in 1952, there was a transition to positive pressure mechanical ventilation via translaryngeal cuffed endotracheal tubes.

Curiass/shell is a shell or a cage which surrounds the chest and is then connected to a portable ventilator. Raincoat or Poncho is a tight fitting suit which is connected through the means of hoses to a portable ventilator. Rocking bed is another method for providing negative pressure ventilation which induces diaphragmatic motion by placement of the patient on a bed which rocks rapidly flat to upright while the contents of abdomen shift. A pneumobelt is a belt with a bladder which can inflate and deflate with air in a cyclic pattern. The diaphgram moves in response to changes in the intraabdominal pressure. Another form of negative pressure ventilation is a pneumowrap.

It was not until the 1980s with the development of nasal masks for continuous positive airway pressure, used for the treatment of obstructive sleep apnea, that there was a renewed interest in NIV and specifically non-invasive positive pressure ventilation.

Principles of NIV: Non-invasive ventilation (NIV) refers to the use of ventilatory methods without the use of an endotracheal tube or a tracheostomy tube which are artificial invasive methods. NIV provides ventilation through the use of a mask of similar device to the patient's upper airway (**Figure 1**). This technique is significantly different from the invasive ones which bypass the upper airway of the patient through the use of a laryngeal mask, tracheal tube or tracheostomy. Initially non-invasive ventilation through the use of masks was used in neuromuscular disorders to provide ventilatory support in the night in view of hypoventilation. This was followed by use of non-invasive ventilation used nocturnally in cases of chronic obstructive pulmonary disease leading to an improvement in the muscle strength of respiratory muscles [1]. Ultimately, NIV delivered through masks turned out to be of utmost benefit and was used as a method of standard ventilation in cases of chronic hypercapnic respiratory failure which could be due to deformities of the chest, neuromuscular disorder or impaired central respiratory drive. Few years later NIV was started to be used in respiratory failure due to lung pathologies rather than respiratory pump failures. Since then, NIV has evolved immensely with a widespread application in the Intensive Care Units.

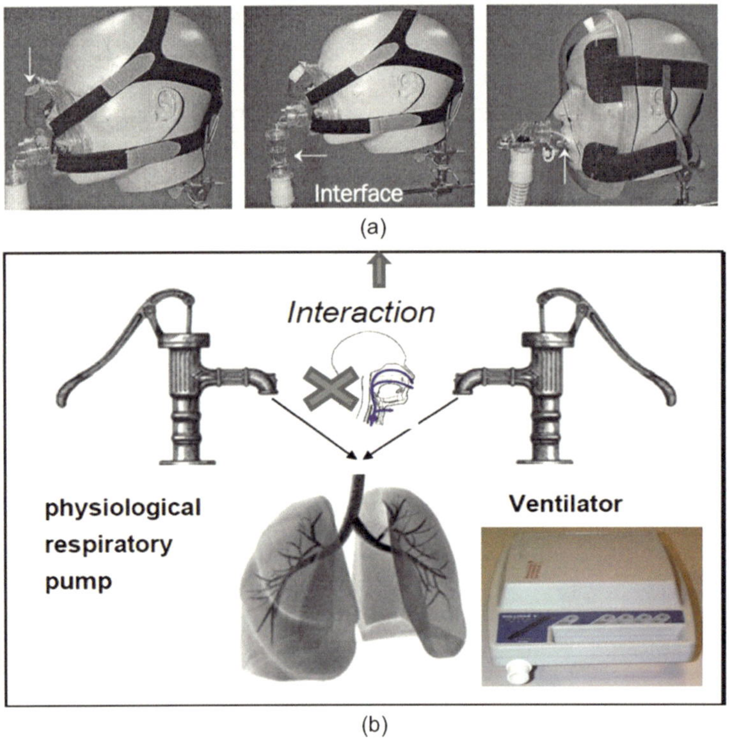


**Figure 1.**
*Principle of NIV is application of any technique to augment alveolar ventilation without use of conduit access to airway and using interfaces at nose, mouth or both to deliver compressed air ± oxygen to lungs to improve efficiency of physiological pump.*

| Advantages | Disadvantages |
|---|---|
| Airway defense mechanism is well preserved | Claustrophobic mask |
| Intermittent use of ventilation | Cannot be used in uncooperative patients |
| Patient is able to eat food (Less chances of hypoglycemia) and communicate properly | Time consuming for the health care staff as gas exchange correction requires time in NIV |
| Physiotherapy can be given easily | No protection of airway |
| Comfortable for the patient when compared to invasive ventilation | Difficult to provide suction as direct access to the bronchial tree is not present |
| Reduced requirement for sedation | Irritation to the eye |
| Avoidance of chances of intubation | Needs to be constantly checked for air leaks |

**Table 1.**
*Showing the advantages and disadvantages of NIV use in intensive care unit.*

Currently NIV is also being used in about 20 to 30 percent of acute hypoxic respiratory failure. NIV has even been used in cases of acute respiratory distress syndrome with an alarming success rate of more than 50 percent with improvement being more predominant in the patients whose oxygenation had improved promptly. The advantages and disadvantages of NIV use in intensive care unit have been shown in **Table 1**.

### 1.1 Interface used in NIV

For the effectiveness of NIV a proper interface is very important, which include variety of masks. These masks include the

- Oronasal or full-face mask,
- Nasal mask,
- Nasal "pillows" consisting of soft pledgets inserted directly into the nostrils,
- Mouthpieces held in place by lip seals resembling a snorkel,
- Total face mask resembling a plastic hockey goalie's mask, and
- The helmet (fits over the entire head).

Advantages and disadvantages of interface -

- Some degree of air leak either through the mouth or around the mask is common however it can be minimized with proper education and cooperation from the.
- The full-face mask interferes with speech, expectoration, and eating and it carries the risks of claustrophobia, aspiration, and rebreathing when compared to the nasal mask.
- Dentures should be left in place to optimize the fitting of the mask.
- The nasal mask requires patent nasal passages and mouth closure to minimize air leaks.

## 2. Modes of noninvasive ventilation

### 2.1 Positive pressure ventilation

Positive pressure ventilation delivers either a tidal volume which is either at a supra-atmospheric pressure or at a preset volume which leads to the inflation of the lungs. Exhalation is itself a passive event; it relies on the elastic recoil of the lungs for the deflation of the lung until equilibrium is attained with the pressure of atmosphere or PEEP.

It is the most commonly utilized mode of NIV in the present time, where the interface with the patient can be in the form of a full face mask, a nasal mask or a nasal pillow.

Benefits of positive pressure ventilation are as follows includes avoidance of intubation and other risks as well as complications which are associated with it. There is also preservation of swallowing along with speech and cough reflex which is beneficial for the patient. There is improvement in the exchange of gas and reduction in the word of breathing through resting of the muscles of respiration.

Candidates for positive pressure ventilation are all the patients with respiratory failure irrespective of the type of respiratory failure and it's type. Patients with acute exacerbation of chronic obstructive pulmonary disease, acute pulmonary edema, pneumonia and exacerbation of bronchial asthma, cystic fibrosis or intrinsic lung disease can be managed with positive pressure ventilation.

Portable ventilators are utilized in order to provide continuous positive airway pressure (CPAP) or BIPAP. CPAP is used to deliver a pressure which is constantly set during inspiration as well as expiration which leads to an increase in the functional residual capacity resulting in improvement of oxygenation, however, it is not strictly a form of ventilatory assistance. Contraindication for the use of positive pressure ventilation is uncooperative patient, patient having a copious amount of secretions where airway protection is not possible, patient with unstable hemodynamics and patients with decreased mental state.

BIPAP is used to provide positive airway pressure in a manner which is biphasic. There is an inspiratory positive airway pressure (IPAP) which is set for inspiration and a lower expiratory positive airway pressure (EPAP) which is set for expiration. Difference obtained from subtracting EPAP from IPAP yields the degree of ventilatory assistance.

EPAP provides a dual benefit by ensuring proper flow in order to flush carbon dioxide from the single tube of ventilator and avoiding rebreathing along with increasing functional residual capacity and opening up the upper airway to prevent apnea as well as hypopnea. It also counterbalances the intrinsic positive end expiratory pressure in patients suffering from chronic obstructive pulmonary disease.

### 2.2 Initiation of NIPPV

A portable ventilator can be used to initiate NIPPV. First, there needs to be setting up of volume targeted strategy and the tidal volumes need to be higher than in invasive ventilation. A tidal volume of 10 to 15 cc/kg is used. This can compensate for the leak of air through the mouth as well as around the mask. Respiratory rate can be decided and chosen as in standard ventilation. Adequacy of ventilation/oxygenation should be checked through the means of arterial blood gas. Tidal volume or respiratory rate can be increased if the minute ventilation needs to be increased. Similarly, in an over ventilated lung, respiratory rate or tidal volume may be decreased. Oxygen supplementation is provided in line with the circuit.

BiPAP uses a pressure targeted strategy for ventilation. Inspiratory pressure or IPAP can be chosen from 8 to 20 cm H2O pressure. It can be thought of as pressure support. As the pressure increases it will be more uncomfortable for the patient. Generally, BiPAP is started between a range of 8 to 11 cm H2O.Expiratory pressure or EPAP is set at 3 to 5 cm H2O.It can be thought of as PEEP. Difference obtained from subtracting EPAP from IPAP is the amount of support being provided to the patient. In case the patient required further ventilation, IPAP level can be increased gradually. A back up rate can be set by the ventilator rate which can be chosen as a value below the patient's spontaneous rate to assure that the patient does not develop apnea. A higher ventilator rate may be chosen in order to prevent periods of prolonged apnea and in order to allow resting of the respiratory muscles. If there needs to be improvement in oxygenation, amount of oxygen can be increased in the circuit or EPAP level may be increased. An Increase in EPAP level leads to decrease in tidal volume. To counter this, IPAP level can be increased in the same increment as the increase in EPAP.

Before Weaning one must consider to check if the patient has improved oxygen saturation at low flow oxygen rate, respiratory rate of below twenty four breaths per minute and ensure that there is interruption of positive pressure ventilation for short duration of time to ensure talking, eating, drinking and assess tolerance and gradually increase these pauses.

Drawbacks in the use of positive pressure ventilation are difficulties arising from the discomfort of the mask, headgear or straps and air leaks. Patients also complain of nasal pain, erythema or breakdown of skin due to use of mask. There can also be nasal congestion or dryness as well as ulceration of the nasal bridge with long duration of mask usage. Eye irritation due to air leak blowing into the eyes, gastric distention and aspiration are other few problems encountered in the use of positive pressure ventilation.

It is important to remember that NIPPV when initiated can induce anxiety in the patients making them uncomfortable. In order to make the patients acclimatized to the technique of NIPPV the patients require a 1:1 assistance by respiratory therapist who also makes fine adjustments in the flow rates and pressures depending on the requirement of the patient. On an average it may take about an hour for patient to become comfortable with NIPPV. IT is crucial to monitor the respiratory rate, heart rate as well as arterial blood gas to detect the effectiveness of NIPPV in correcting acute respiratory failure. At any point, if the patient deteriorated on NIPPV, conversion to endotracheal tube in order to ensure proper oxygenation should be considered.

## 3. Negative pressure

*Ever since the development of positive pressure nasal and face interfaces, negative pressure is not used commonly.*

Negative pressure ventilation works of the mechanism of delivering pressure which is sub-atmospheric resulting in the expansion of the chest and air being drawn into the lungs through the nose and mouth. When the pressure which is around the chest wall returns to normal pressure of the atmosphere there shall be passive expiration. Negative pressure ventilation endeavors to mimic normal breathing mechanics.

Methods for providing negative pressure ventilation include iron lung which was used primarily in the epidemic of polio in the era of 1950's.Curiass/shell is a shell or a cage which surrounds the chest and is then connected to a portable ventilator.

Raincoat or Poncho is a tight fitting suit which is connected through the means of hoses to a portable ventilator. Rocking bed is another method for providing negative pressure ventilation which induces diaphragmatic motion by placement of the patient on a bed which rocks rapidly flat to upright while the contents of abdomen shift. A pneumobelt is a belt with a bladder which can inflate and deflate with air in a cyclic pattern. The diaphgram moves in response to changes in the intraabdominal pressure. Another form of negative pressure ventilation is a pneumowrap.

Indications for negative pressure ventilation include chronic respiratory failure secondary to neuromuscular disease- polio, muscular dystrophy. Generally used for nocturnal ventilatory support, with the patient breathing spontaneously during the day. Negative pressure ventilation has also been used in acute respiratory failure, there are 2 different studies which examined the use of the iron lung and poncho wrap (respectively) in COPD patients with acute respiratory failure. Both studies demonstrated the effectiveness of negative pressure ventilation to correct CO2 retention.

Drawbacks encountered with negative pressure ventilation are worsening of obstructive sleep apnea, problems with correct fitting as well as portability issues. Attendants are often required for the application and removal of the device making the process troublesome for the patients. For the use of negative pressure ventilation the patients must sleep in supine position only making it difficult to use.

## 4. NIV in acute hypoxemic respiratory failure

Respiratory failure is one of the most common cause leading to admission in intensive care unit and is the concluding pathway of a wide range of diseases with differing pathophysiologies.

A mechanism-based approach enables the clinician to identify the most likely cause for the respiratory failure and to treat appropriately.

### 4.1 Types of respiratory failure

A. Hypercapnic respiratory failure - Ventilatory failure and is recognized by an elevated PaCO2 above normal. Patient usually have respiratory pump failure with lungs which are normal or ventilatory failure as a consequence of airway disease or extremely severe lung parenchymal disease with normal lungs or as a consequence of airways disease or very severe parenchymal lung disease.

B. Hypoxemic respiratory failure - Failure of gas exchange is characterized as hypoxemia (PaO2 less than 60 mm Hg), with or without the widening of gradient between the alveoli and artery. Most of the patients suffering from this type of respiratory failure have a shunt physiology or mismatch of ventilation-perfusion (V/Q) as the primary mechanisms of hypoxemia. Most of these patients have abnormalities detected on chest x-ray.

C. Mixed respiratory failure with multiple components of various pathophysiologies which can result in hypoxemia as well as hypercarbia.

D. Type 4 respiratory failure occurs in patients who are postoperative having normal lungs with normal respiratory pump who are either sedated or paralyzed or have metabolic demands which exceed the patient's ability to compensate. This is seen commonly in patients suffering from intensive metabolic abnormalities such as metabolic acidosis or sepsis.

#### *4.1.1 Acute hypoxemic respiratory failure*

Main component is The alveolar–arterial oxygen gradient = PAO2 – PaO2. The normal value is between 10 and 15 mm Hg and is influenced by age, i.e. increases by approximately 3 mm Hg every decade after the age of 30 years. For an FiO2 = 21%, it should be 5 to 25 mm Hg and for an FiO2 = 100%, it should be <150 mm Hg. Hypoxemic respiratory failure with a widened alveolar–arterial oxygen gradient is caused by V/Q mismatching or shunt pathophysiology. Hypoxemia due to V/Q mismatch improves with supplemental oxygen, while no improvement in cases with shunt.

Disease which result in the flooding of airspace, complete or partial collapse of the lung, pulmonary vascular abnormalities or airway disease are the common source of hypoxemic respiratory failure.

Principles for managing the patients suffering from hypoxemic respiratory failure mainly include:-

- Rapid re-establishing of optimal arterial saturation which commonly necessitates the need of intubation and mechanical ventilation.

- By and large, the patients having infiltrates in the lungs respond less well to non-invasive ventilation.

- Using optimal amount of positive end-expiratory pressure ensures the reduction of FiO2 levels to non-toxic levels (FiO2 less than 60 percent).

- Using a strategy with low tidal volume along with permissive hypercapnia in patients suffering from acute respiratory distress syndrome or acute lung injury.

- Providing general supportive care to the patient in the intensive care unit while there is resolution of patient's pulmonary pathology.

#### *4.1.2 Causes*

A. Due to increased alveolar arterial gradient with V/Q mismatch

- Airway disease- Chronic Obstructive Pulmonary Disease, Asthma, Cystic Fibrosis, Bronchiolitis Obliterans Syndrome

- Interstitial lung disease- Interstitial Pulmonary Fibrosis, Sarcoidosis, Interstitial pneumonia e.g. Covid 19 pneumonia

- Alveolar filling – Pulmonary Edema, Left heart failure, Acute Lung Injury/ Acute Respiratory Distress Syndrome, Pneumonia, Trauma, Contusion, Alveolar hemorrhage/proteinosis, Transfusion Related Acute Lung Injury, Acute interstitial pneumonitis, Acute eosinophilic pneumonia, Bronchiolitis Obliterans Organizing Pneumonia/Cryptogenic Organizing Pneumonia, Aspiration, Upper airway obstruction, Near drowning

- Pulmonary vascular disease – Thromboembolism, Fat embolism

B. Due to increased alveolar arterial gradient with Shunt

- Same as causes of alveolar filling
- Atelactesis – Post operative, Immobility
- Intra pulmonary vascular shunt- Pulmonary arteriovenous malformation, Hepatopulmonary syndrome
- Intracardiac shunt – Patent foramen ovale, Atrial septal defect, Ventricular septal defect

*4.1.3 Evidences of NIV in acute hypoxemic respiratory failure*

Oxygen to improve hypoxia in acute hypoxic failure appears to be standard of care and in 2005 it was shown that NIV is better than oxygen in improving PaO2/FiO2 by unloading of respiratory muscles [2]. In Earlier studies it was shown when used appropriately NIV is as effective as invasive mechanical ventilation in improving PaO2/FiO2 by Antonellii et al. thereby avoiding all complications related to endotracheal intubation and related ventilation [3]. But the most important aspect of success versus failure of NIV in acute hypoxic respiratory failure is 'Timing of initiation vis a vis progression of inciting disease as well as severity of respiratory failure" [4]. In Acute Hypoxic Respiratory Failure, NIV needs to be initiated for mild to moderate hypoxia and before the disease has progressed (a) as window of opportunity to use NIV is narrow (b) as once disease has progressed IMV is indicated.

Failure of NIV in acute hypoxic respiratory failure needs to be identified early to prevent higher mortality. Meta-analysis of NIV use in ALI/ARDS showed intubation rate of 46% (30–86%) and mortality of 35% (19–69%) and these widely variable results indicate that different diseases states causing hypoxic respiratory failure as well as baseline characteristics of individual patients along with threshold of intubation of the centre contribute to success or failure of NIV [5]. But studies are clear that milder is the hypoxia, lesser are the chances of failure indicating baseline PaO2 is one of the determinant of NIV outcome [6]. Further studies also showed earlier is the better as disease has potential for reversibility. Immunosuppressed patients also showed good success rates with use of NIV in acute hypoxic respiratory failure [7]. Hence, use of NIV in acute hypoxic respiratory failure is indicated as follows [8]:

Level 1: in acute cardiogenic pulmonary edema as well as immunocompromised patients with acute hypoxic respiratory failure.

Level 2: evidence is to use in post-operative hypoxic respiratory failure, COPD with community acquired pneumonia as well as to prevent hypoxic failure in acute severe asthma. However NIV in severe community acquired pneumonia without any underlying comorbidity to support use of NIV needs to be used with caution as in to prevent Extubation failure. Also in patients with do not intubate or resuscitate orders.

Level 3: in patients with thoracic trauma, upper respiratory tract obstruction, partial upper airway obstruction as well as treatment in acute severe asthma but with caution to use in severe ARDS.

Level 4: In very elderly (>75 years), obesity hypoventilation syndrome and in IPF with caution.

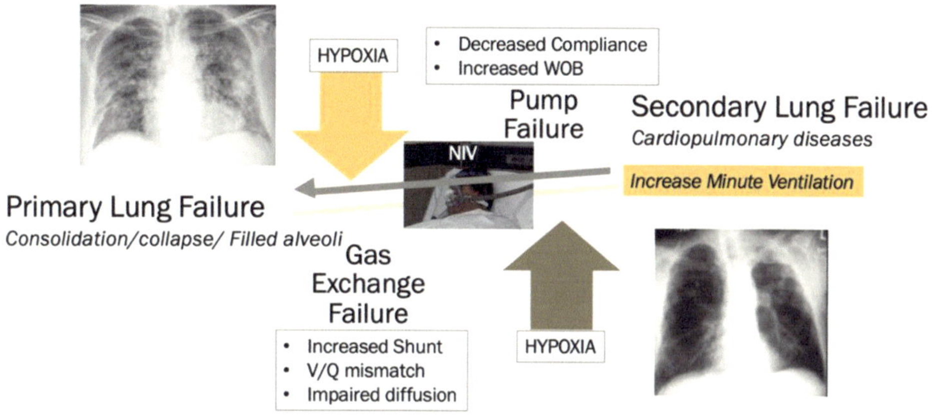


**Figure 2.**
*Rationale of using NIV in acute hypoxic respiratory failure.*

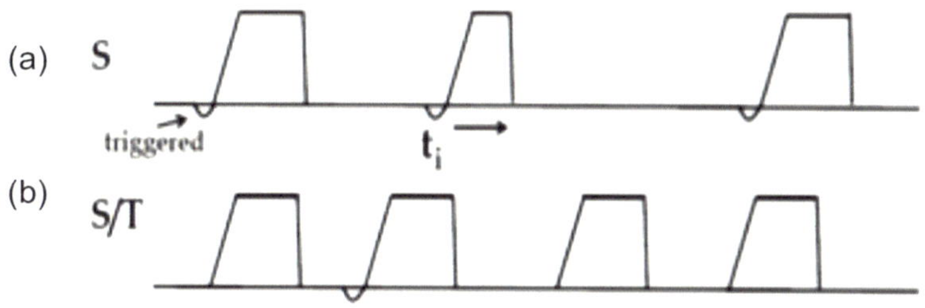


**Figure 3.**
*Showing modes of bi-level NIV used in hypoxic respiratory failure (spontaneous and spontaneous timed).*

Rationale of using NIV in acute hypoxic respiratory failure is that the primary or secondary lung failure, both lead to acute hypoxia which can be either due to abnormality in the exchange of gas or failure of the respiratory pump which leads to increase in minute ventilation, this is reversed by the use of NIV (**Figure 2**).

Modes of bi-level NIV used in hypoxic respiratory failure are defined by triggering: S-Spontaneous (a. patients efforts only triggering NIV), S/T- Spontaneous timed (b. patient's own as well as timed triggering to give back up RR in case patient has irregular and slow breathing pattern to safe guard adequate ventilation, misses a breath (**Figure 3**).

Helmet ventilation is the most secure form of NIV in severely hypoxic patients but claustrophobia may prohibit its use. It can be used in severe hypoxic respiratory failure and it's use in Covid 19 pneumonia and ARDS showed favorable results vis a vis oxygen therapy. However, cardiac instability is contraindication.

NIV is also used to support interventional procedures in patients with hypoxia while doing bronchoscopy or transesophageal Echocardiography.

However, in contrast to use of NIV in hypercapnic respiratory failure in hypoxic respiratory failure one needs to look beyond lungs into systemic component of disease process e.g. shock, acidosis, multi organ failure, etc. as these situations will favor invasive mechanical ventilation.

70% of failures of NIV occur within 48 hours, indicating need for intensive monitoring and identifying features of early failure proactively (**Figure 4**).

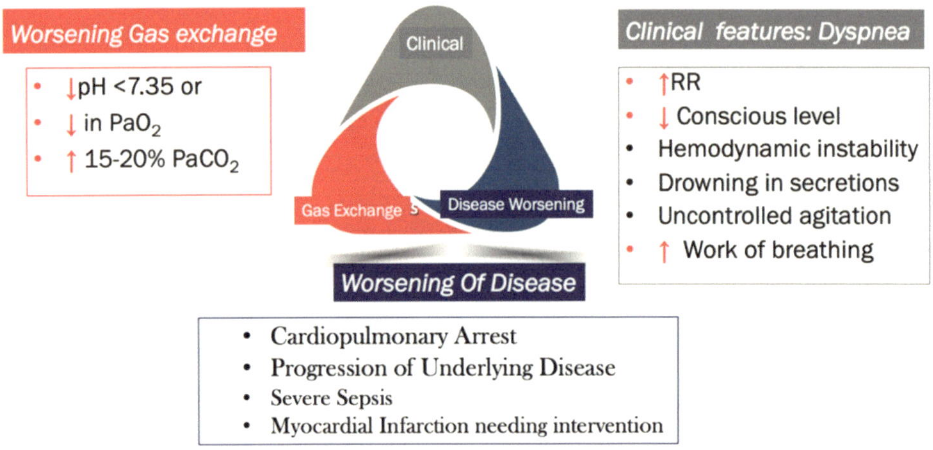


**Figure 4.**
*Identify failing NIV early by bedside monitoring worsening of clinical features, gas exchange parameters and primary disease causing hypoxia.*

It has been shown that delaying intubation in such cases increases mortality and adds no benefit. Most common cause of failure is inability to correct hypoxia in 2/3rd of failed NIV's followed by intolerance, progression of disease with hemodynamic instability. Changing NIV machine to guaranteed volume mode (AVAP's or iVAP) can help to improve tidal volume and hypoxia. Hence all such cases should be managed in ICU settings only. Intolerance can be managed by using different types of masks or correcting into leaks. Use of sedation is strictly under observation with full facility and readiness to intubate.

NIV has penetrated deeply into the roots of medical management even in rural health facilities of India where a study conducted in rural India concluded that [9]:

- NIV is able to reduce the mortality and endotracheal intubation through the improvement of the outcome of patients.

- NIV in selected group of patients is the modality of treatment of acute hypoxemic respiratory failure.

- Close monitoring should be ensured to depict the patient's response in order to take the decision of intubation on time.

- Early introduction of NIV can help in the reduction of intubation rates and the subsequent complications as well as nosocomial infections associated with intubation.

## 5. NIV in COVID-19 pneumonia

Covid 19 pandemic caused devastation across the world with hospitalization in 5–15% and 5% requiring ICU due to severe and critical hypoxic failure. Secondary to severe covid pneumonia and ARDS. NIV has been used from the beginning of pandemic with China reporting NIV works well and results were similar to that of HFNC in Covid 19. They also reported no nosocomial outbreaks of Covid 19 infection in health cares in ICU units which used NIV. Europe started using CPAP with variable success rates as well as concerns. Initial reports of NIV use in Covid 19 showed that CPAP trial succeed in 40% when used in those requiring >15 L/min of O2 by non-rebreathing mask with baseline $SpO_2/FiO_2$(SFR) of >110, RR > 30/min and NLR > 8. Repeat SFR at 30–120 min improved in all patients but cut off of SFR 180 was the best predictor of success or failure of CPAP trial but patients who failed had high mortality (38%) [10]. Intubation rates and mortality in Covid 19 patients who received NIV was similar to the group which received HFNC. European Respiratory Society Living Guideline for management of Covid 19 has recommended use of NIV with helmet or full face mask to treat acute hypoxic respiratory failure secondary to coronavirus infection provided there is no immediate indication for IMV [11]. But caution must be exercised in close monitoring to identify signs of NIV failure in Covid pneumonia. There have been reports of full recovery in COVID-19 patients even after extensive lung involvement by judicious noninvasive ventilation strategies linked with prone ventilation [12–14].

## 6. High flow nasal cannula

Keeping in mind the human factors of comfort, humidification and warming of inspired air are essential in creating an effective oxygenation system (**Figure 5**). Basic components of high flow nasal cannula (HFNC) include a flow generator providing gas flow rates up to 60 liters per minute, an air-oxygen blender that achieves escalation of FIO2 from 21–100% irrespective of flow rates, and a humidifier that saturates the gas mixture at a temperature of 31 to 37 C [15]. To minimize condensation, the heated humidified gas is delivered via heated tubings through a wide-bore nasal prong. In this system all settings are controlled independently, so maximum delivery of oxygen thence better outcome.

Mechanism responsible for high efficacy includes Physiological dead space (which accounts for approximately one-third of the tidal volume of breathing) washout of waste gasses including carbon dioxide (CO2), Decreased respiratory rate, Positive end-expiratory pressure, Increased tidal volume and Increased end-expiratory volume.

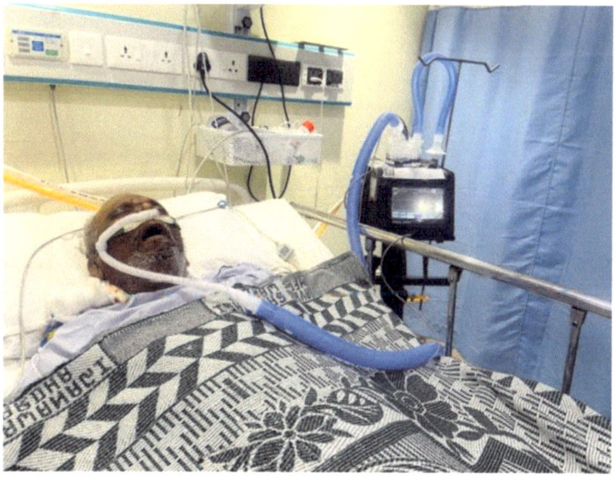

**Figure 5.**
*Showing high flow nasal cannula used for hypoxic respiratory failure.*

**Advantage:**

- It creates a positive end-expiratory pressure to the lower airways in addition to providing positive pressure support to the nasopharynx.
- It applies a splinting force to keep alveolar airways from collapsing under increased surface tensile stresses during exhalation.
- This allows for improved alveolar recruitment, increasing the effective available surface area within the lungs for gaseous diffusion both to and from the blood.
- It has taken over low-flow nasal cannula as later blows cool, dry air directly into the nasal passages which leads to drying of the mucosa, irritation, epistaxis, and cracking of the tissue barriers. This causes, uncomforted and restlessness in the patients thence poor adherence to therapy.
- Now a days high-flow nasal cannula systems are having inbuilt warming and humidification systems which provides humidified and body temperature air that is non-irritating to the mucosa, increasing patient comfort.

There is increasing evidence of clinical application of HFNC in Acute hypoxemic respiratory failure, Post-surgical respiratory failure, Acute heart failure/pulmonary edema, Hypercapnic respiratory failure, COPD, Pre and post-extubation oxygenation, Obstructive sleep apnea, Do not intubate the patient and so on.

## 7. Conclusions

Hence, Non-Invasive Ventilation (NIV) is a useful tool for pulmonary diseases including acute hypoxic respiratory failure which has penetrated deeply into the routes of India with a vast scope of usage and advantages. A proper monitoring while the patient is on NIV ensures early pick up of NIV failure helping in the proceeding of appropriate corrective steps.

## Conflict of interest

"The authors declare no conflict of interest."

## Author details

Dhruv Talwar[1], Sunil Kumar[2]* and Deepak Talwar[3]

1 Department of Medicine, Jawaharlal Nehru Medical College, Datta Meghe Institute of Medical Sciences (Deemed to be University), Wardha, Maharashtra, India

2 Post Graduate Department, Jawaharlal Nehru Medical College, Datta Meghe Institute of Medical Sciences (Deemed to be University), Wardha, Maharashtra, India

3 Metro Centre for Respiratory Diseases, Noida, Uttar Pradesh, India

*Address all correspondence to: sunilkumarmed@gmail.com

## References


[1] Ali MS, Talwar D, Singh M. P229 nocturnal noninvasive ventilation improves muscle strength in stable COPD patients with respiratory failure. Thorax. 2012;**67**:A165

[2] L'Her E, Deye N, Lellouche F, Taille S, Demoule A, Fraticelli A, et al. Physiologic effects of noninvasive ventilation during acute lung injury. American Journal of Respiratory and Critical Care Medicine. 2005;**172**(9):1112-1118

[3] Antonelli M, Conti G, Rocco M, Bufi M, De Blasi RA, Vivino G, et al. A comparison of noninvasive positive-pressure ventilation and conventional mechanical ventilation in patients with acute respiratory failure. The New England Journal of Medicine. 1998;**339**(7):429-435

[4] Nava S, Navalesi P, Conti G. Time of non-invasive ventilation. Intensive Care Medicine. 2006;**32**(3):361-370

[5] Agarwal R, Aggarwal AN, Gupta D. Role of noninvasive ventilation in acute lung injury/acute respiratory distress syndrome: A proportion meta-analysis. Respiratory Care. 2010;**55**(12):1653-1660

[6] Zhan Q, Sun B, Liang L, Yan X, Zhang L, Yang J, et al. Early use of noninvasive positive pressure ventilation for acute lung injury: A multicenter randomized controlled trial. Critical Care Medicine. 2012;**40**(2):455-460

[7] Hilbert G, Gruson D, Vargas F, Valentino R, Gbikpi-Benissan G, Dupon M, et al. Noninvasive ventilation in immunosuppressed patients with pulmonary infiltrates, fever, and acute respiratory failure. The New England Journal of Medicine. 2001;**344**(7):481-487

[8] Nava S, Hill N. Non-invasive ventilation in acute respiratory failure. Lancet. 2009;**374**(9685):250-259

[9] Bajaj A, Kumar S, Inamdar AH, Agrawal L. Noninvasive ventilation in acute hypoxic respiratory failure in medical intensive care unit: A study in rural medical college. International Journal of Critical Illness and Injury Science. 2019;**9**(1):36-42

[10] Noeman-Ahmed Y, Gokaraju S, Powrie DJ, Amran DA, El Sayed I, Roshdy A. Predictors of CPAP outcome in hospitalized COVID-19 patients. Respirology. 2020;**25**(12):1316-1319

[11] Chalmers JD, Crichton ML, Goeminne PC, Cao B, Humbert M, Shteinberg M, et al. Management of hospitalised adults with coronavirus disease 2019 (COVID-19): A European Respiratory Society living guideline. The European Respiratory Journal. 2021;**57**(4):2100048

[12] Jain A, Talwar D, Kumar S. Spectrum of respiratory involvement in COVID 19 era; an overview. Indian Journal of Forensic Medicine & Toxicology. 2020;*14*(4):6593-6599

[13] Shah P, Mahajan S, Kumar S, Acharya S, Vohra M, Bagga C, et al. Severe COVID-19 case with HRCT score of 25/25: A survival story. Journal of Pharmaceutical Research International. 2021;**33**(46B):148-153

[14] Halani D, Jaiswal A, Kumar S, Talwar D, Madaan S. Post natal COVID-19 induced severe acute respiratory distress syndrome managed with monoclonal antibody and prone ventilation. Medical Science. 2021;**25**(112):1427-1431

[15] Segovia B, Velasco D, Jaureguizar Oriol A, DíazLobato S. Combination therapy in patients with acute respiratory failure: High-flow nasal cannula and non-invasive mechanical ventilation. Archivos de Bronconeumología (Engl Ed). 2019;**55**(3):166-167

Chapter 3

# Renal Replacement Therapies in the Intensive Care Unit

*Dominic Godbout, Philippe Lachance and Jean-Maxime Côté*


## Abstract

Renal replacement therapies (RRT) are commonly used in critically ill patients to achieve solute clearance, maintain acid-base status, and remove fluid excess. The last two decades have seen the emergence of large randomized control trials bringing new evidence regarding how RRT should now be managed in the ICU. RRT is considered a vital supportive care and needs to be adequately prescribed and delivered. This chapter first summarizes the basic principles and characteristics of the three major RTT modalities: intermittent hemodialysis (IHD), prolonged intermittent RRT (PIRRT), and continuous RRT (CRRT). Then, the large body of literature regarding indications for initiation (*early* vs *late*), choice of modality (*intermittent* vs *continuous* and *diffusion* vs *convection*), dosing (*intensive* vs *less-intensive*), and anticoagulation alternatives is reviewed to guide clinical decision-making. Recent evidence in the optimal timing of discontinuing RRT is reported. Finally, troubleshooting scenarios frequently seen in clinics and requiring an adapted RRT prescription are also discussed.


**Keywords:** renal replacement therapy, intermittent hemodialysis, hemofiltration, continuous renal replacement therapy, prolonged intermittent renal replacement therapy, intensive care unit

## 1. Introduction

Prevalence of acute kidney injury (AKI) was evaluated at 22% in hospital settings in a large meta-analysis of 3.5 million patients and raised up to 57% when admitted to intensive care units (ICUs) [1, 2]. The incidence of dialysis-requiring AKI has increased by 10% yearly from 2000 to 2009 in the United States [3]. Hence, renal replacement therapy (RRT) is widely used in modern acute care settings as a supportive management of severe acute kidney injury (AKI) and multiorgan failure (MOF). While RRT in chronic end-stage kidney disease (ESRD) is mostly reserved for nephrologists, its prescription in context of acute-care settings is shared between many medical specialties.

The first section reviews the basic principles and characteristics of the different modalities used in ICUs nowadays. Then, the main section is meant to guide clinicians in evidence-based RRT prescribing by examining the most relevant body of literature published in the last decade. Indications, timing of initiation, modality choice, dosing, anticoagulation, and discontinuing RRT are discussed. Finally, some specific and more challenging scenarios are briefly covered as well as other pragmatic aspects.

## 2. Basics

### 2.1 Principles: diffusion, ultrafiltration, and convection

Despite major improvements in technologies from the first experimental hemodialysis (HD) in 1924 to the first continuous arteriovenous hemofiltration (CAVH) circuit in 1977, general principles guiding the removal of water and solutes for almost any type of extracorporeal renal replacement therapies initiated in the ICU remain the same: diffusion, convection, ultrafiltration and sometimes adsorption (see **Figure 1**) [4]. These three major concepts will be integrated according to the renal replacement therapy (RRT) modality chosen. The notable exception is peritoneal dialysis (PD), which, nowadays, is rarely initiated in acute setting such as AKI in ICU adult populations. However, PD for AKI is often used in children and has been shown useful in resource-limited settings (e.g., no reliable access to electricity or CRRT devices) as well as in extraordinary circumstances when usual CRRT capacities have been overflowed (e.g., recent COVID19 pandemic). Nevertheless, in most centers, PD as a modality of RRT is restricted to ESRD patients requiring maintenance dialysis and is rarely an option in ICUs. For these reasons, only blood-based extracorporeal renal replacement therapies will be reviewed in this Chapter.

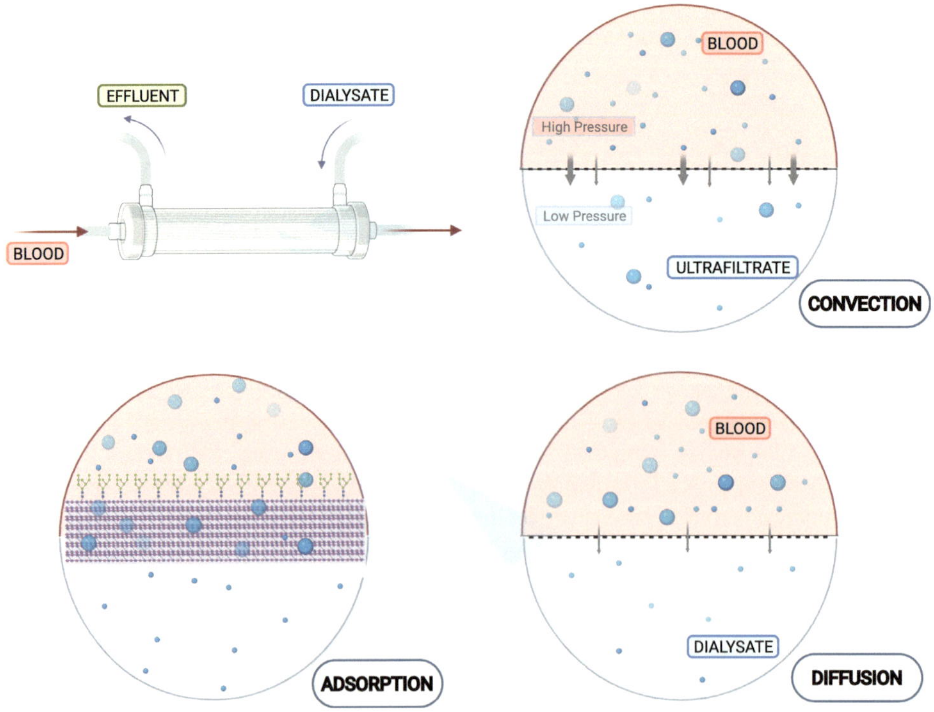


**Figure 1.**
*Principles guiding blood-based extracorporeal RRT.*

**Diffusion**, as used in HD, is the movement of solutes across a semipermeable membrane. The direction and intensity of that movement are driven by the concentration gradient (from higher to lower). Circulating blood and the dialysate in opposite direction on each side of the semipermeable membrane (countercurrent flow) maximizes concentration gradient and potentiates solute clearance. Another key aspect driving diffusion-based clearance is the size of the solute, where smaller solutes (<100 Daltons) cross the membrane faster than larger molecules. Other important properties are protein binding, distribution volume, and electrical charge [5].

**Ultrafiltration** (UF) is the movement of fluid across a semipermeable membrane using pressure differential (from higher to lower pressure) to generate the ultrafiltrate. In RRT, net UF represents the total amount of fluid removed to obtain the net fluid balance, which can be prescribed per hour (e.g., −50 mL/h) during CRRT or per session (e.g., −2 liters) during intermittent HD.

**Convection**, as used in hemofiltration, is the clearance of dissolved solutes along plasma crossing the semipermeable membrane (ultrafiltrate) (a mechanism sometimes called "solvent drag"). When used alone, convection requires to generate a large amount of ultrafiltrate (containing dissolved toxins/solutes) to achieve adequate clearance. Hence, a substantial amount of sterile solution needs to be reinjected to the patient to compensate for the volume removed by convection to maintain volume and solutes homeostasis. Convection can remove larger, middle-sized molecules at which diffusion is inefficient [5, 6].

**Adsorption** is the adherence of a molecule to the surface of a polymer, or a charged membrane exposed to the blood. As opposed to convection, where middle and small molecules completely cross the membrane and are therefore removed by the effluent fluid, the polymer/membrane will be progressively saturated by those molecules, leading to a progressive reduced adsorptive capacity for longer treatments. There is an increasing interest in the potential of adsorption to reduce the inflammatory response by adsorbing cytokines, endotoxins, or exotoxins mostly in septic shock. Mixed results on the true added benefit of this technology have been reported and dialyzer/cartridge generating adsorption is not widely used in the current practice [7].

### 2.2 Modalities characteristics: IHD, PIRRT/SLED, and CRRT

All extra-corporeal RRT technologies used in ICUs can be separated into three modalities: intermittent hemodialysis (IHD), prolonged intermittent RRT (PIRRT) (also called sustained low-efficiency dialysis [SLED]), and continuous RRT (CRRT). Their ability in fluid and solute removal is all based on one or on the combination of the basic principles described above (See **Figure 2**).

In HD (A) and CVVHD (B), blood and dialysate circulate on each side of the semipermeable membrane. Diffusion is the driving force that contributes to solute clearance. For all RRT devices, pressure differential between the two compartments, using dedicated pumps to generate transmembrane pressure (TMP), controls convection flow and ultrafiltration rate. The removed liquid containing waste is usually called effluent for all modalities.

In CVVH (C), convection is the main mechanism used to provide solute clearance. The generation of ultrafiltrate is continuously compensated by the reinjection of replacement fluid. That replacement can be injected before the filter, after the filter, or a combination of both (called pre- vs. post-filter reinjection ratio). Adding pre-filter replacement fluid dilutes blood and its components, notably its hematocrit reducing the overall thrombogenicity. Hence, increasing pre-filter/post-filter ratio reduces the risk of circuit clotting. On the opposite, a proportional increase in hematocrit at the end of the filter will occur when increasing the convection volume in a 100% post-filter CVVH configuration.

CVVHDf (D) results from the combination of (B) and (C) where both convection and diffusion achieve solute clearance. The replacement fluid may be mixed pre- and post-filter as well in addition to using a countercurrent dialysate flow. However, diluting blood pre-filter also decreases the concentration gradient, which is a major driving force in diffusion. The prescription should be adapted according.

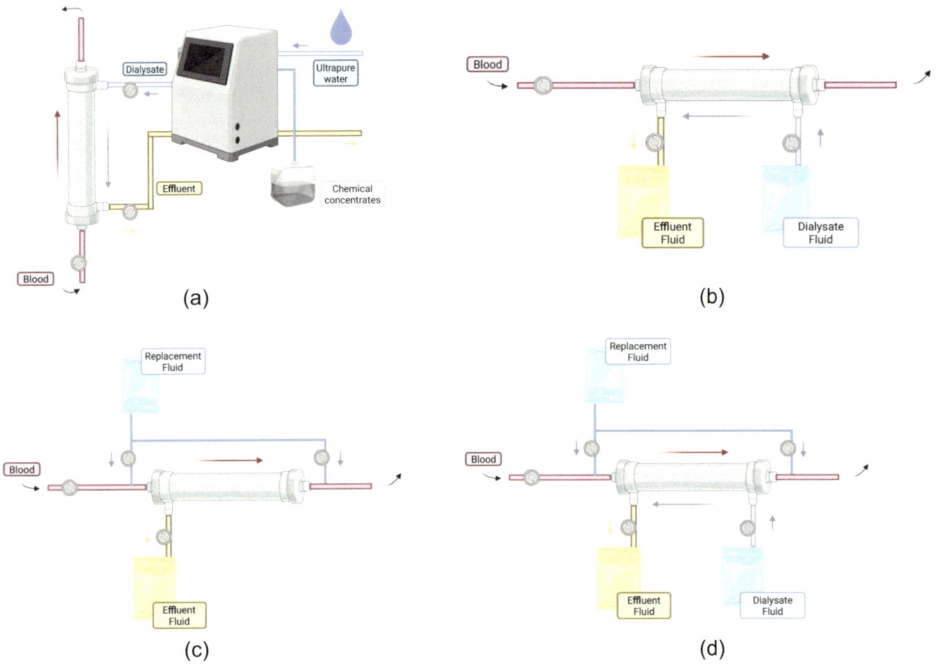


**Figure 2.**
*Schematic representation of IHD and CRRT circuits' configuration. (A) HD: A dedicated intermittent HD device generates large volumes of physiological dialysate using sterile water and chemical concentrates. Up to 800 mL/min of new dialysate can be constantly generated for most HD devices. The composition/prescription of this dialysate can be individualized according to the patient's need. (B)(C)(D) a dedicated CRRT machine uses commercially available bags of physiological solution, using low effluent flow (20–35 mL/kg/h).*

Net fluid balance (net UF) can be obtained in all modalities: in IHD and CVVHD, by generating a TMP, which leads to ultrafiltrate. In CVVH and CVVHDF, the volume of reinjection needs to be slightly lower than the ultrafiltrate generates, which leads to a negative fluid balance.

It should be noted that some centers can generate high volumes of convection when using intermittent RRT. This modality is named hemodiafiltration (HDF), requires an adapted dialysis machine, and is increasingly used in Europe and Asia for ESRD patients. However, its implementation in ICU settings remains limited, partly due to the need to maintain a water treatment system adapted to HDF [8]. As a result, when reporting intermittent RRT in the ICU, we generally consider only IHD.

From a clinical standpoint, each modality is associated with typical blood flow rates (Qb) and dialysate flow rates (Qd) which translates into conventional treatment durations and frequencies (see **Table 1**).

PIRRT represents the application of intermittent hemodialysis technology (machine, filter, dialysate) with a modification of the typical IHD prescription. The objective is to provide a better hemodynamic tolerability than IHD. Hence, in centers offering this modality, PIRRT is generally used in place of CRRT such as in patients with hemodynamic instability, especially if a substantial negative fluid balance (net UF rate) is desired. PIRRT is typically delivered 8 hours with slower blood and dialysate flows than IHD. However, this modality is not optimal for acute RRT indication such as severe hyperkalemia or intoxication with dialyzable substances (e.g., salicylates, methanol, and ethylene glycol) because of its lower flow rates. In some centers, a dedicated HD nursing staff is required to deliver a PIRRT treatment.

| | Intermittent hemodialysis (IHD) | Prolonged intermittent renal replacement therapy (PIRRT) | Continuous renal replacement therapy (CRRT) |
|---|---|---|---|
| **Type of clearance**<br>D=Diffusion<br>C=Convection | IHD: D<br>HD*f*: D + C | SLED: D<br>SLED*f*: D + C | CVVH: C<br>CVVHD: D<br>CVVHD*f*: D + C |
| **Type of machine** | IHD machine | Usually, IHD machine | CRRT machine |
| **Duration** | 3–4 hours | 6–12 hours | Continuous |
| **Frequency** | 3–4 days/week | 3-7 days/week | Continuous |
| **Qb range (mL/min)** | 350–400 | 150–250 | 100–250 |
| **Qd range (mL/min)** | 500–800 | 100–300 | 25–30 |
| **Usual UF rate** | 0–5000 mL/ session | 0–5000 mL/session | 0–200 mL/hour |

*IHD: intermittent hemodialysis, HDf: intermittent hemodiafiltration; SLED: sustained low-efficiency dialysis, SLEDf; sustained low-efficiency hemodiafiltration.*

**Table 1.**
*Typical prescribing patterns of RRT modalities.*

CRRT is characterized by small flow rates, notably reinjection, dialysis, and UF rates. It allows reducing the hemodynamic effects of fluid and solute changes. However, this continuous modality requires a permanent connection to the CRRT machine, supervision and is at high risk of clotting if no anticoagulation is prescribed. In most centers, an adequately trained ICU nurse can manage a CRRT treatment.

## 3. Prescribing RRT

Even though RRT is widely used, and most ICUs have elaborated standardized protocols to simplify IHD/CRRT prescription, many factors need to be considered before, during, and when stopping this therapy: patient's characteristics, local resources, physician's preferences as well as scientific evidence.

### 3.1 Initiating

#### *3.1.1 Indications*

Indications for initiating RRT in acute care are frequently classified as *absolute* vs. *relative* or as *emergent* vs. *semi-urgent*. Although the terms "absolute" or "emergent" might seem dichotomic as if a clear cut-off was defined, they are subject to interpretation in clinical practice [9]. It is generally accepted to begin RRT in a timely manner once any of these conditions occur if concordant with the goals of care (see **Table 2**).

On the other hand, whether to initiate and when to do so while not meeting any of these indications has received a lot of interest in the last few years in the attempt to prevent morbidity and mortality. Indeed, initial observational studies had supported the rationale that a proactive/early RRT will help to quickly normalize renal homeostasis while minimizing inflammation and uremic toxicity. On the other hand, this approach could lead to initiate RRT in patients who will never develop clear indications as some will spontaneously recover in addition to exposing them to unnecessary

| |
|---|
| 1. Refractory to medical treatment:<br>a. Hypervolemia with pulmonary edema<br>b. Severe hyperkaliemia ($K^+$ > 6.5 mmol/L) or rapidly rising kaliemia<br>c. Severe acidemia (pH <7.1–7.2) due to metabolic acidosis ($HCO3^-$ < 12–15 mmol/L) |
| 2. Uremic complications of renal failure (e.g., pericarditis and encephalopathy) |
| 3. Dialyzable toxin exposure |

**Table 2.**
*Absolute indications of initiating RRT.*

RRT complications. This has led to the constantly evolving *early* vs. *late* paradigm which has been investigated in five recent landmark randomized controlled trials (RCTs) (see **Table 3**). A careful reminder of the definitions used to classify severity of acute kidney injury (AKI) is mandatory before reviewing these trials (see **Table 4**).

In 2016, the results of the first large RCT trying to answer this complex question were published. The Early Versus Late Initiation of Replacement Therapy In Critically Ill Patients with AKI (**ELAIN**) trial was a single-center based in Germany with mostly surgical patients [12]. The RRT modality was CVVHDF at a dosing of 30 ml/kg/h and using regional citrate as anticoagulation. All participants in the early group (< 8 h of stage 2) vs. 91% in the delayed group (< 12 h of stage 3 or $K^+$ > 6 mmol/L, urea >100 mg/dL, $Mg^{2+}$ > 4 mmol/L, UO < 200 ml/12 h or refractory edema) received RRT. An important characteristic is a relatively small difference in the time to begin RRT from initial randomization across groups (21 hours (IQR 18–24)) and in the overall use of RRT (9%) between both arms. A significant statistical mortality benefit was obtained favoring the early arm (HR 0.66 (0.37–0.97), p = 0.03). A few months later, the Artificial Kidney Initiation in Kidney Injury (**AKIKI**) trial was published; a multicenter and much larger study from 31 French ICUs totalizing 620 patients [13]. The modality was at the discretion of physicians (30% received CRRT as sole therapy) and 80% had sepsis-related conditions (sepsis, severe sepsis, or septic shock). Almost all participants in the early group (< 6 h of stage 3) compared to 51% in the delayed group ($K^+$ > 6.0 mmol/L, urea>112 mg/dL, pH < 7.15, pulmonary edema or oliguria/ anuria >72 h) received RRT. The difference in the time to begin RRT between the two arms was 55 hours. No difference was seen in mortality (60 days), but more catheter-related bloodstream infections were reported in the early group (p = 0.03). In 2018, the Initiation of Dialysis Early Versus Delayed in the Intensive Care Unit (**IDEAL-ICU**) trial, which took place in 29 ICUs in France was published [14]. This trial included 488 patients within the first 48 hours of their septic shock. The modality was also at the discretion of physicians. Almost all participants in the early group (< 12 h of Failure stage) compared to 62% in the delayed group ($K^+$ > 6.5 mmol/L, pH < 7.15, pulmonary edema or persistent AKI 48 h after inclusion) received RRT. No difference was seen in mortality (90 days). It is important to notice that this trial was stopped early for futility (initially designed for 864 patients).

In an attempt to definitively clarify the question of *Timing*, the Standard versus Accelerated Initiation of RRT in AKI (**STARRT-AKI**) trial was later published in 2020. It included 3019 patients from 168 ICUs in 15 countries [15]. Patients mostly received CRRT (70%) and had both medical (65%) and surgical (35%) conditions. Almost all participants in the early group (*accelerated strategy*) (<12 h of stage ≥2) compared to 62% in the delayed group (*standard strategy*) ($K^+$ > 6 mmol/L, pH < 7.2, $HCO3^-$ < 12, pulmonary edema or persistent AKI 72 h after inclusion) received RRT. Once again, no difference was seen in mortality (90 days), including in the subgroup

| **Studies (year)** | **Settings** | **Population** | **Early-group criteria** | **Delayed-group criteria** | **Primary outcome** | **Secondary outcomes or safety endpoints** |
|---|---|---|---|---|---|---|
| ELAIN (2016) | Germany single center CVVHDF (30 ml/kg/h) | n = 231 93.5% surgical (46.8%-cardiac) SOFA 15.6 vs. 16.0 | < 8 h of stage 2 RRT: 100% | < 12 h of stage 3 or $K^+ > 6$ mmol/L, *urea >100 mg/dL, $Mg^{2+} > 4$ mmol/L, UO < 200 ml/12 h, refractory edema RRT: 91% | 90-day mortality: E: 39.3% D: 54.7% HR 0.66 (0.37–0.97, **p = 0.03**) | Median RRT duration (days): E: 9 vs. D: 25 HR:0.69 (0.48–1.00) 90-day RRT requirement: OR 0.87 (0.31–2.44) |
| AKIKI (2016) | France 31 ICUs 30% CRRT-only >50% intermittent | n = 620 80% sepsis-related SOFA 10.9 vs. 10.8 | < 6 h of stage 3 RRT: 98% | $K^+ > 6.0$ mmol/L, urea>112 mg/dL, pH < 7.15, pulmonary edema or oliguria/anuria >72 h RRT: 51% | 60-day mortality: E: 48.5% D: 49.7% (p = 0.79) | 60-day RRT dependence: E: 2% vs. D: 5% (p = 0.12) CRBI: E: 10% vs. D:5% **(p = 0.03)** |
| IDEAL-ICU (2018) | France 29 ICUs stopped early (futility) CRRT and IHD | n = 488 <48 h of septic shock SOFA 12.2 vs. 12.4 | < 12 h of Failure stage (RIFLE) RRT: 97% | K+ > 6.5 mmol/L, pH < 7.15, pulmonary edema or persistent AKI after 48 h RRT: 62% | 90-day mortality: E: 58% D: 54% (p = 0.38) | Median RRT duration (days): E: 4 vs. D: 2 90-day RRT dependence: E: 2% vs. D: 3% (p = 1.00) |
| STARRT-AKI (2020) | 15 countries 168 ICUs 70% CRRT 30% intermittent | n = 3019 65% medical 35% surgical SOFA 11.6 vs. 11.8 | <12 h of stage ≥2 RRT: 97% | $K^+ > 6$ mmol/L, pH < 7.2, $HCO3^- < 12$, pulmonary edema or persistent AKI 72 h after inclusion RRT: 62% | 90-day mortality E: 43.9% D: 43.7% (p = 0.92) | Median RRT duration (days): E: 4 vs. D: 5 RR = −0.48 (−0.82–(−)0.14) 90-day RRT dependence: E: 10% vs. D: 6% RR = **1.74** (95% CI 1.24–2.43) Any adverse event: E:23% vs. D:16.5% **(p < 0.001)** |
| AKIKI-2 (2021) | France 39 ICUs 40% CRRT 60% intermittent | n = 278 55% septic shock For inclusion (3/3): 1)MV or vasopressor 2)AKI stage 3 3)Oligo-anuria >72 h or urea 112 to 140 mg/dL | <12 h of fulfilling inclusion criteria RRT: 98% | $K^+ > 6$ mmol/L, pH < 7.15, *urea>140 mg/dL, pulmonary edema (No time criteria) RRT: 79% | RRT free days (day 28) E:12 D: 10 (p = 0.93) | 60-day mortality: E:44% vs. D:55% (p = 0.07) RRT duration (days) E:5 vs. D: 5 (p = 0.75) 60-day RRT dependence: E:4% vs. D: 1% (p = 0.62) |

**Urea conversion to SI units: 100 mg/dL = 35.7 mmol/L, 112 mg/dL = 40 mmol/L, 140 mg/dL = 50 mmol/L.*
*E: Early-group, D: Delayed-group, UO: urine output, CRBI: Catheter-related bloodstream infection, MV: mechanical ventilation.*

**Table 3.**
*Landmark RCTs on timing of RRT initiation.*

| KDIGO (2012) [10] | | | RIFLE (2007) [11] | | |
|---|---|---|---|---|---|
| **Stage** | **Creatinine** | **Urine output** | **Stage** | **Creatinine** | **Urine output** |
| 1 | 1.5–1.9 x baseline<br>Or<br>≥ ↑ 0.3 mg/dL | < 0.5 ml/kg/h x 6–12 h | **Risk (R)** | 1.5 x baseline<br>Or<br>↓ GFR > 25% | < 0.5 ml/kg/h x 6 h |
| 2 | 2.0–2.9 x baseline | < 0.5 ml/kg/h x ≥ 12 h | **Injury (I)** | 2 x baseline<br>Or<br>↓ GFR > 50% | < 0.5 ml/kg/h x 12 h |
| 3 | ≥ 3.0 x baseline<br>Or<br>≥ 4.0 mg/dL<br>Or<br>Initiation of RRT | < 0.3 ml/kg/h x ≥ 24 h<br>Or<br>Anuria ≥12 h | **Failure (F)** | 3 x baseline<br>Or<br>↓ GFR > 75%<br>Or<br>≥ 4.0 mg/dL | < 0.3 ml/kg/h x ≥ 24 h<br>Or<br>Anuria ≥12 h |
| | | | **Loss (L)** | Persistent acute renal failure >4 weeks | |
| | | | **ESKD (E)** | ESKD >3 months | |

*↑: increase of serum creatinine, ↓: decrease of GFR, ESKD: end-stage kidney disease.*
*Creatinine conversion to SI units: 0.3 mg/dL = 26.8 μmol/L; 4.0 mg/dL = 353.6 μmol/L).*

**Table 4.**
*KDIGO and RIFLE classifications of AKI.*

analysis (including medical vs. surgical). Notably, a difference was obtained in RRT dependence at 90 days which was higher in the accelerated group (RR = 1.74 [95% CI 1.24–2.43]). Significantly more adverse events (23% vs. 16.5% $p < 0.001$) occurred when exposed to the accelerated strategy, mainly driven by hypotension ($p < 0.001$), and mild hypophosphatemia ($p < 0.001$), with the trend toward more bloodstream infections ($p = 0.07$). Compared to previous studies, distinctive pragmatic characteristics should be noted. First, if the clinician did not have absolute equipoise regarding initiation of RRT (e.g., expected impending renal recovery), the patient was not included. Also, the delayed strategy did not mandate RRT initiation once the criteria were fulfilled but was based on clinical judgment. Results from this study have substantially affected how and when RRT is now initiated in ICUs worldwide.

STARRT-AKI has confirmed evidence against the preemptive use of RRT prior to developing standard RRT initiation criteria. However, a question remained unanswered: how far can we delay RRT initiation without negative outcomes? The Artificial Kidney Initiation in Kidney Injury-2 (**AKIKI-2**) trial, published in 2021, was developed to answer that question, assessing the potential benefits of a more-delayed strategy in terms of RRT-free days. That trial took place in 39 ICUs in France and included 278 patients. To be eligible for randomization, three criteria had to be achieved: (1) mechanical ventilation or vasopressor + (2) AKI stage 3 + (3) Oligo-anuria >72 h or urea 112 to 140 mg/dL[1]. Almost all participants in the "early group" (similar to the *delayed group* from STARRT-AKI) (<12 h of fulfilling inclusion criteria) compared to 79% in the delayed group (*more-delayed strategy*) ($K^+ > 6$ mmol/L, $pH < 7.15$, urea>140 mg/dL[2], pulmonary edema) received RRT. Median time between randomization and initiation of RRT was 3 hours versus 33 hours. Noteworthy, the difference in RRT use of 19% between the two groups is about half of what

[1] Urea criteria led to inclusion of 61% in the *delayed* and 55% in the *more-delayed* strategy.

[2] Urea criteria led to initiation of RRT in 59%.

has been obtained in the three previous studies. No difference was reported in RRT-free days on day 28 even though no time criteria were applied in the delayed group, contrasting to previous studies. The primary outcome of 60-day mortality was not significantly higher in the more-delayed group compared to delayed (55% vs. 44%, p = 0.07). Though, in the preplanned multivariate analysis, the more-delayed strategy was associated with increased 60-day mortality (HR 1.65 p = 0.018). Overall, the more-delayed strategy did not demonstrate decreased use of RRT, but worrisome findings suggesting potential harms.

#### *3.1.2 Predicting the need of RRT*

As shown in those studies where a substantial number of patients randomized to a delayed strategy never required RRT initiation, correctly predicting who will progress to an AKI stage where RRT is required is complex in a real-life setting. Since the last decade, a growing number of tools and biomarkers have been developed, and reported useful, to inform about the likelihood a patient with AKI will worsen, and progress to receive RRT [16]. Various urine and blood biomarkers have been studied, such as the urine neutrophil gelatinase-associated lipocalin (uNGAL), interleukin-18 (IL18), or the NephroCheck (TIMP2*IGFBP7), with a pooled AUC or 0.720, 0.668 and 0.857 respectively. More functional biomarkers, such as a diuretic response of less than 200 mL to a loading dose of 1.0 to 1.5 mg/kg of intravenous furosemide (FST – Furosemide stress test) have also been shown useful in predicting the risk of progression to RRT with a pooled sensitivity and specificity of respectively 0.84 (95% CI 0.72–0.91) and 0.77 (95% CI 0.64–0.87) [17]. The growing interest in such complementary tools is associated with the publication of multiple confirmation studies in recent years, leading to recent consensus in favor of their use in standard clinical practice [18]. However, their implementations in real-life ICU settings are still in the beginning.

#### *3.1.3 Conclusion*

In summary, only the first smallest single-center RCT of almost entirely surgical patients has shown a mortality benefit of early initiation of RRT compared to a delayed strategy. The three subsequent trials consisting of more than four thousand patients with a variety of modalities and populations (including surgical subgroup analysis) concluded the absence of such advantages of early initiation. Also, the added resources required to initiate 35–45% more RRT must not be neglected. Furthermore, significant harms have been reported in the early-initiation approach: catheter-related bloodstream infections (AKIKI), 90-day RRT dependence, and any adverse event (STARRT-AKI). On the other hand, the latest trial might help in determining the upper limit of postponing RRT. Therefore, a conservative approach consisting of watchful waiting, unless a life-threatening indication emerges, seems recommended for most cases with the caveats that the risk-benefits ratio is uncertain once criteria used for inclusion in the latest trial are reached.

### 3.2 Modality choice

#### *3.2.1 Intermittent vs. continuous*

Although there are substantial variations in practice, hemodynamic instability is the most common reason to choose slow intermittent (PIRRT) or continuous (CRRT)

| Study (year) | Design | # of Pts | CRRT | IHD | Survival | Renal Recovery |
|---|---|---|---|---|---|---|
| Mehta et al. (2001) *ARF ICU* | RCT | 166 | CVVHDF or CAVHDF | Qb 200–300 | CRRT 34.5% IHD 52.4% **($p < 0.02$)** | CRRT 34.9% IHD 33.3% (p = NS)* |
| Guerin et al. (2002) | Prospective observational (unadjusted) | 587 | variable | variable | CRRT 20.6% IHD 41.2% **($p < 0.001$)** | Not mentioned |
| Gasparovic et al. (2003) | RCT | 104 | CVVH | Qb 200–250 | CRRT 28.8% IHD 40.4% (p = NS) | Not mentioned |
| Augustine et al. (2004) | RCT | 80 | CVVHD | Qb 300 | CRRT 32.5% IHD 30.0% (P=NS) | CRRT 12.5% IHD 10.0% (p = NS)* |
| Vinsonneau et al. (2006) *HEMODIAFE* | RCT | 259 | CVVHDF | Qb 278 | CRRT 32.6% IHD 31.5% ($p = 0.98$) | CRRT 93.3% IHD 90.2% (p = NS)** |
| Lins et al. (2009) *SHARF Trial* | RCT | 316 | CVVH | Qb 100–300 | CRRT 41.9% IHD 37.5% ($p = 0.430$) | CRRT 74.5% IHD 83.1% ($p = 0.474$)** |
| Schefold et al. (2014) *CONVINT Trial* | RCT | 252 | CVVH | Qb 200–250 | CRRT 45.4% IHD 39.7% ($p = 0.72$) | CRRT 77.2% IHD 73.6% ($p = 0.90$)** |
| Truche et al. (2016) | Prospective observational (adjusted) | 1360 | CVVH or CVVHD | variable | CRRT 53.5% IHD 65% (p = NS) | CRRT 64.7% IHD 42.9% ($p = 0.29$)** |

**In all patients randomized.*
***In patients who survived at ICU discharge.*
*CAVHDF: Continuous arteriovenous hemodiafiltration, p: p-value, NS: Non-significant.*

**Table 5.**
*Major studies comparing CRRT to IHD.*

therapy. The 2012 KDIGO AKI guidelines suggest using CRRT rather than intermittent RRT for these patients (grade B – moderate quality of evidence) [19]. However, empirical data has not proven what might seems obvious at first to clinicians. In fact, the use of PIRRT or CRRT compared to IHD in randomized trials has failed to demonstrate differences in hard outcomes such as mortality or recovery of renal function [20–26] (see **Table 5**). Still, it is important to note that heterogeneity is found in dosing, CRRT subtypes, delivered blood flow, and that the most unstable patients were excluded for most of them.

As mentioned earlier, in patients with hemodynamic instability, the choice between PIRRT and CRRT mostly depends on local availability. The level of evidence regarding PIRRT is still limited, but advantages compared to CRRT may include: reduced costs and flexible treatment schedule allowing the patient to be more easily mobilized during daytime. As opposed to fixed CRRT solutions, the dialysate composition can be more easily adapted to the patient's needs even during the dialysis session. However, no clear antimicrobial dose adjustments are recommended with that modality. In patients who regain stability, the RRT prescription can be rapidly adapted, from PIRRT to a conventional IHD prescription, using the same technology.

### *3.2.2 Diffusion vs. convection*

Given that both clearance methods are efficient at clearing small solutes, the question is mainly about the added benefit (or harm) of removing medium-sized pro-inflammatory molecules such as cytokines, endotoxins, or exotoxins. In ESRD patients, for those treated with HDF compared to IHD, some benefits were demonstrated in large RCTs on reducing intradialytic hypotension and use of erythropoietin-stimulating agents, but more importantly, an all-cause mortality benefit (HR 0.78, 95%CI 0.62–0.98) and cardiovascular mortality (HR0.69, 95%CI 0.47–1.0) were obtained when optimal convective volumes were delivered [27]. However, in AKI no such benefits have been demonstrated with certainty. A 2012 meta-analysis of 19 RCTs, comparing hemofiltration (CVVH) to hemodialysis (mostly CVVHD) found no effect on mortality (RR 0.96, 95%CI 0.71–1.15), or other clinical outcomes (RRT dependence in survivors, vasopressor use, organ dysfunction) despite increased clearance of medium to larger molecules, including inflammatory cytokines [28]. Despite fewer studies, similar results have been shown when comparing intermittent modalities offering diffusion only (IHD) to convection (HDF) in ICUs [8].

### *3.2.3 Conclusion*

Since neither the modality mode (*intermittent* vs. *continuous*) nor the clearance method (*convection* vs. *diffusion* vs. both) has shown its superiority, local expertise remains a core element when choosing the modality. Pragmatical aspects such as required staff, costs, and immobilization consequences on the ability to perform rehabilitation and anticoagulation are also important considerations, all summarized in **Table 6**.

## 3.3 Dosing

Like any treatment, RRT intensity or delivered dose must be tailored to the patient's need. While underdosing may result in insufficient clearance of uremic toxins, uncontrolled electrolytes, or acid–base status, overdosing leads to electrolytes disorders, hydrophilic micronutrients depletion, hazardous therapeutics dosing (e.g., antibiotics), and unnecessary expenses [29]. Ultrafiltration is a critical component of RRT prescribing but is not part of *dosing* which refers to the clearance capability. Another key point is that the actual delivered dose is often lower than the prescribed dose for multiple reasons: vascular access limiting Qb, interruptions for radiologic studies or surgery, circuit change or clotting, etc.

### *3.3.1 Intermittent modalities*

For all intermittent modalities, as seen in **Table 7**, the blood flow rate is the limiting factor highlighting the value of maximizing the potency of vascular access. A subsequent option to optimize clearance is increasing the *frequency* or *duration* of treatments. Then, to lesser levels, increasing filter surface and dialysate flow rate[3]. For dosing assessment (or *clearance adequacy*), guidelines recommend using the clearance

[3] A Qd/Qb ratio higher than 1.5 has minimal to no impact on small solute clearance while using high-flux filter

| Modality | | | Anticoagulation* |
|---|---|---|---|
| IHD | Flow | High (Qb < Qd) | Without<br>± saline flush<br>± heparin-coated filters<br>Systemic:<br>UFH (continuous)<br>LMWH (bolus) |
| | + | Short sessions – Allow exams and mobilization<br>Lowest cost<br>Lowest immobilization | |
| | — | Hypotension with rapid fluid removal<br>Higher complexity (dedicated dialysis staff) | |
| | HDF<br>-Removal of medium-sized molecules (added benefit uncertain in AKI)<br>-Large amount of replacement fluid requiring ultra-pure water (Dedicated water treatment complicating ICU implementation) | | |
| CRRT | Flow | Low Qd and convection, Moderate Qb | Without<br>Systemic: UFH<br>Regional: citrate |
| | + | Hemodynamic stability<br>No treatment-induced increase intracranial pressure<br>Fine fluid control<br>Lower complexity to operate (ICU staff only) | |
| | — | Hypothermia – Negative energetic balance<br>Immobilization<br>Higher costs (commercial bag for replacement fluids) | |
| PIRRT | Flow | moderate (Qb ≥ Qd) | Without<br>± saline flush<br>± heparin-coated filters<br>Systemic: UFH, LMWH |
| | + | Online production of dialysate and IHD tubing (lower cost than CRRT)<br>Reduced immobilization (low rehabilitation impact if done overnight) | |
| | — | Higher complexity (dedicated dialysis staff in some centers) | |

*Qb: blood flow rate, Qd: dialysis flow rate, UFH: unfractionated heparin, LMWH: Low-molecular-weight heparin.*
**See anticoagulation section for more details.*

**Table 6.**
*Pragmatical considerations with RRT modalities.*

of urea over the treatment session. It can be estimated with the urea reduction ratio (URR)[4] and the $Kt/V_{urea}$[5] for small molecules clearance, while the appreciation of medium-sized molecules removal is inferred by the quantification of beta-2-microglobulin (not done in acute care RRT) [19, 30–32]. However, variations of urea generation and difficulty defining the distribution volume ($V_{urea}$) in metabolically unstable patients are serious limitations in acute care settings. While KDIGO-AKI 2012 guideline still recommends an overall $Kt/V_{urea}$ of 3.9 per week (1A – high-quality), the European Renal Best Practice (ERBP) 2013 position statement recommends against the use of $Kt/V_{urea}$ as a measure of dialysis (1A – high-quality) but

---

4 URR = 100 × (1 - [$C_t/C_o$]), in which $C_t$ = BUN at the end of dialysis and $C_o$ = predialysis BUN

5 $Kt/V_{urea}$, in which K = clearance, t = time, V = distribution volume estimated as body water volume. For example, Qb 300 ml/min x 180 min = 54,000 ml = 54 L and 70 kg x 0.6 L/kg (60% body weight) = 42 L. Estimated non-adjusted $Kt/V_{urea}$ = 54/42 = 1.3

More refined equation using pre/post-dialysis BUN is now used to account for UF and physiological BUN generation, known as the Daugirdas equation.

| Studies (year) | Settings | Strategy | | Dose delivered (Kt/V or total effluent rate ± SD) | Mortality | Secondary outcomes or safety endpoints |
|---|---|---|---|---|---|---|
| ATN (2008) | USA 27 ICUs n = 1124 AKI due to ATN | **Less-intensive** | | | 60-day mortality: L: 51.5% I: 53.6% (p = 0.47) | Hypotension requiring vasopressor L: 10% vs. I: 14% (p = 0.02) Electrolyte disturbance L:20.7% vs. I:25.6% (p = 0.05) |
| | | | IHD/SLED 3x/week | 1.31 ± 0.33 | | |
| | | | CVVHDF 20 mL/kg/h | 22.0 ± 6.1 | | |
| | | **Intensive** | | | | |
| | | | IHD/SLED 6x/week | 1.32 ± 0.36 | | |
| | | | CVVHDF 35 ml/kg/h | 35.8 ± 6.4 | | |
| RENAL (2009) | Australia & New Zealand 35 ICUs n = 1508 AKI | **Less-intensive** | | | 90-day mortality: L: 44.7% I: 44.7% (p = 0.99) | Hypophosphatemia L: 54% vs. I: 65% |
| | | | CVVHDF 25 mL/kg/h | 22.7 ± 17.8 | | |
| | | **Intensive** | | | | |
| | | | CVVHDF 40 mL/kg/h | 33.4 ± 12.8 | | |

*AKI: acute kidney injury; ATN: acute tubular necrosis; L: Less-intensive group, I: Intensive group.*

**Table 7.**
*Landmark RCTs on RRT dosing strategy.*

rather to ensure that intermittent therapy is adapted to maintain volume balance and metabolic homeostasis [19, 33].

One RCT includes intermittent modalities compared to dosing-based strategies. The Acute Renal Failure Trial Network **(ATN)** study included 1124 patients in 27 centers in the United States and compared intensive-therapy (IHD or SLED 6 days/week if stable and CVVHDF 35 mL/kg/h if unstable) to less-intensive therapy (IHD or SLED 3 days/week if stable and CVVHDF 20 ml/kg/h if unstable) [34]. Targeted $Kt/V_{urea}$ was 1.2 to 1.4 for intermittent therapy and additional UF-only session could be done in the less-intensive strategy. No difference was obtained in 60-day mortality, RRT duration, or recovery of kidney function. More hypotension and electrolyte disturbance were seen in the intensive strategy.

### *3.3.2 Continuous modalities*

For CRRT, as the trans-membrane equilibrium is almost achieved at the end of the filter for small solutes, the limiting factor for clearance is therefore the effluent flow rate. Hence, the total delivered effluent rate, normalized to actual weight, is used to quantify clearance. According to the circuit configuration, that total effluent rate corresponds to the sum of the reinjection flow (pre- and post-filter) (if CVVH or CVVHDF) + the rate of dialysate flow (CVVHD or CVVHDF) + UF (see **Figure 3**). Even if the UF rate is included in the equation of the delivered dose, in clinical practice it is added once the targeted dose has been prescribed. First, it usually

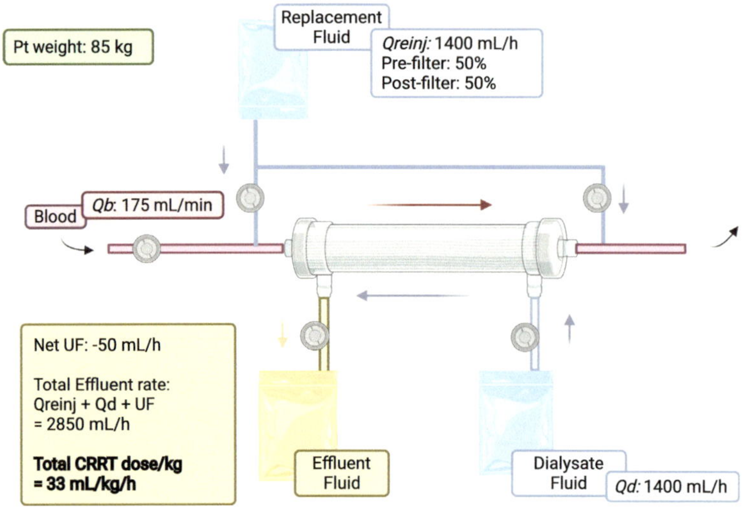


**Figure 3.**
*Example of CRRT dosing using a CVVHDF circuit.*

represents a fraction of total effluent in an average size patient.[6] Also, since this rate is regularly modified, its exclusion always allows minimally sufficient delivered dose. Other options to optimize CRRT clearance such as increasing blood flow rate or filter surface have a reduced effect on optimizing clearance efficiency.

Between 2000 and 2008, four major RCTs evaluated the impact of different CRRT doses in critically ill patients. In 2000, using CVVH in 425 patients, three groups were compared [20 vs. 35 vs. 45 (mL/kg/h)] and mortality was significantly higher in the lowest UF rate group at 15 days after stopping RRT [35]. No difference was reported between the two higher rates. In 2002, using CVVH in 106 patients, three groups were compared [early high-volume (48.2 mL/kg/h) vs. early low-volume (20.1 mL/kg/h) vs. late low-volume (19.0 mL/kg/h)] and no mortality benefits was seen at 28 days [36]. In 2006, a study of 206 patients compared two groups [CVVH (25 mL/kg/h) vs. CVVHDF (reinjection rate 25 mL/kg/h + dialysis rate 18 mL/kg/h)] and mortality was significantly higher in the CVVH-only (at 28-day and three months) [37]. In 2008, using CVVHDF in 254 patients [20 vs. 35 (mL/kg/h)] and no mortality benefit was detected [38].

To confirm these previous findings from single-center trials, two multicenter RCTs (USA and AUSNZ) focused on this topic (see **Table 7**). In 2008, the **ATN** study reported no advantage in regards to mortality, duration of RRT, or recovery of kidney function. In 2009, the Randomized Evaluation of Normal Versus Augmented Level Replacement Therapy (**RENAL**) study, with more than 1508 patients from 35 ICUs in Australia and New Zealand and using CVVHDF with post-filter reinjection randomized participants between higher (40 mL/kg/h) vs. lower (25 mL/kg/h) intensity group [39]. As in the ATN study, no difference in mortality was observed. Based on these results, the KDIGO-AKI guideline recommends a delivered effluent volume of at least 20–25 mL/kg/h for AKI patients requiring RRT (1A – high-quality). As previously mentioned, a slightly higher dose should be prescribed in order to achieve that

[6] In an 80 kg patient, an UF of 100 mL/h on a total dose of 25 ml/kg/h (2000 mL/h) represents 5%.

target regarding the dose truly delivered [19]. Some situations may require greater rates such as extreme metabolic imbalances or acute liver failure (see *Clinical Pearls* section).

#### *3.3.3 Conclusion*

In summary, for both modalities, current evidence does not support using intensive therapy for all patients. For intermittent modalities, it seems appropriate to prescribe IHD at least 3 times a week to maintain volume and metabolic balance as long as there is no sign of underdosing (either a $Kt/V_{urea} < 1.2$ per session or URR $< 67\%$). The weekly $Kt/v_{urea}$ does not apply in patients requiring additional IHD sessions to achieve a volume balance, as well as in patients with significant renal function. For continuous therapies, a prescribed effluent volume of 25–30 mL/kg/h is adequate in most scenarios to ensure a delivered dose of at least 20–25 mL/kg/h.

### 3.4 Anticoagulation

Sustained circuit patency is crucial to optimize delivered RRT and contact of blood with extracorporeal circuit activates platelets and pathways of coagulation [40]. KDIGO-AKI guidelines suggest a flow chart to guide anticoagulation decision [19]. At first, it integrates the risk–benefit ratio of anticoagulation and whether another condition requiring systemic anticoagulation is present. RRT can be performed without or with systemic or regional anticoagulation.

#### *3.4.1 No anticoagulation*

Although KDIGO-AKI guideline recommends using anticoagulation when bleeding risk is low, it is still common practice in many centers to deliver RRT without anticoagulation in this scenario unless filter patency is an issue. For example, in the STARRT-AKI trial, 24% of the 3019 included patients had no anticoagulation at the initiation. A key concept in preventing circuit clotting is maintaining a low filtration fraction (FF). Filtration fraction indicates relative fluid removed from blood across the dialysis membrane. Higher percentage means higher concentration of blood constituents. Fractions above >20% are associated with increased clotting [41]. The equation for CRRT (blood flow rate being converted from mL/min to mL/h to standardize units) is:

$$FF = \frac{\text{Total UF rate}}{(\text{Plasma flow} + \text{Pre} - \text{filter})\text{ rates}} = \frac{(\text{pre} - \text{filter} + \textbf{total UF} + \textbf{post} - \textbf{filter})\text{ rates}}{((1 - \textbf{hematocrit})\text{x } \textbf{blood flow}\text{ ml/h x 60 min/h}) + \text{Pre} - \text{filter})\text{ rates}}$$

*where **total UF** usually integrates all intravenous volumes received by the patient (e.g., IV medications, IV fluids, parenteral nutrition) in addition to the net UF (negative volume balance targeted) converted to mL per hour.*

Modifying elements only found to either the numerator or the denominator (marked in bold) have higher impact on the FF. Hence, from a clinical perspective, reducing FF is achievable by modifying flow rates: reduce net UF, increase pre-filter/post-filter ratio, increase blood flow, reduce hematocrit. Additionally, since hematocrit might be reduced by pre-filter reinjection, it is obvious that administering blood transfusion directly pre-filter should be avoided when possible. Also, the catheter patency is essential by allowing prescribed flow rates, by avoiding stasis induced by alarms (e.g., kinked) and by maintaining a laminar flow (right jugular or femoral access).

For intermittent therapies, major assets helping prevent clotting are shorter sessions and higher blood flows, but clotting may be seen even if using heparin-coated filters, especially when substantial UF volume is removed. If convection is used (HDF or SLEDf), pre-filter reinjection can be used as well.

*3.4.2 Systemic*

Most used agents are unfractionated heparin (UFH) and low-molecular-weight heparins (LMWH). Mostly reserved for patients with heparin-induced thrombocytopenia (HIT), direct thrombin inhibitors (e.g., argatroban and bivalirudin) or Xa inhibitors (e.g., fondaparinux and danaparoid) have been used in intermittent and continuous therapies, but will not be discussed further [42, 43].

UFH has some advantages (e.g., short half-life, antagonist readily available, low costs, and a large experience), but has substantial drawbacks (e.g., narrow therapeutic, unpredictable kinetics and heparin resistance, HIT) [19]. Thrombocytopenia is frequently encountered in ICU occurring in up to 44% of patients. However, HIT remains relatively uncommon in critically ill patients, with a reported incidence from 0.2–5% [44], and has been reported with intermittent and continuous RRT. When used solely for circuit anticoagulation, both the loading and infusion UFH doses need to be adapted to the patient's bleeding/clotting risk as well as continuously monitored with aPTT.

LMWH has replaced UFH in most dialysis units (intermittent therapies) mainly because of convenience of a single dose at start of session associated with the same efficacy (at preventing circuit thrombosis) and security (bleeding) [45]. In addition, a more reliable response is obtained (no monitoring required) along with a reduced risk of HIT. LMWH has been used for CRRT with monitoring of anti-Xa levels [46], but longer half-life and risk of accumulation combined with incomplete reversal by protamine may limit widespread use.

*3.4.3 Regional*

When systemic anticoagulation is not warranted by another indication than maintaining RRT circuit, regional anticoagulation is the recommended strategy. Regional heparinization has been described in CRRT (combining pre-filter UFH, and post-filter protamine), but KDIGO recommends against its use, notably in patients with increased bleeding risk [19]. Likewise, use of regional citrate anticoagulation (RCA) has been evaluated in intermittent therapies [47] but is not common practice. Hence, emphasis will be placed on RCA in CRRT.

As demonstrated in **Figure 4**, RCA may be perceived as complex [48] but has undeniable advantages: no risk of HIT, lower risk of bleeding compared to UFH along with longer filter lifespan. It is therefore recommended as first line for anticoagulation in CRRT in KDIGO-AKI guideline if no contraindication [19]. A 2015 meta-analysis demonstrated reduced circuit loss compared to UFH [HR 0.76 (95%CI 0.50–0.98) for systemic and HR 0.52 (95%CI 0.35–0.77) for regional] and reduced bleeding [RR 0.36 (95%CI 0.21–0.60)] [49]. A 2020 German RCT of 638 patients in 26 centers demonstrated longer filter lifespan (47 vs. 26 hours, $p < 0.001$), no mortality difference

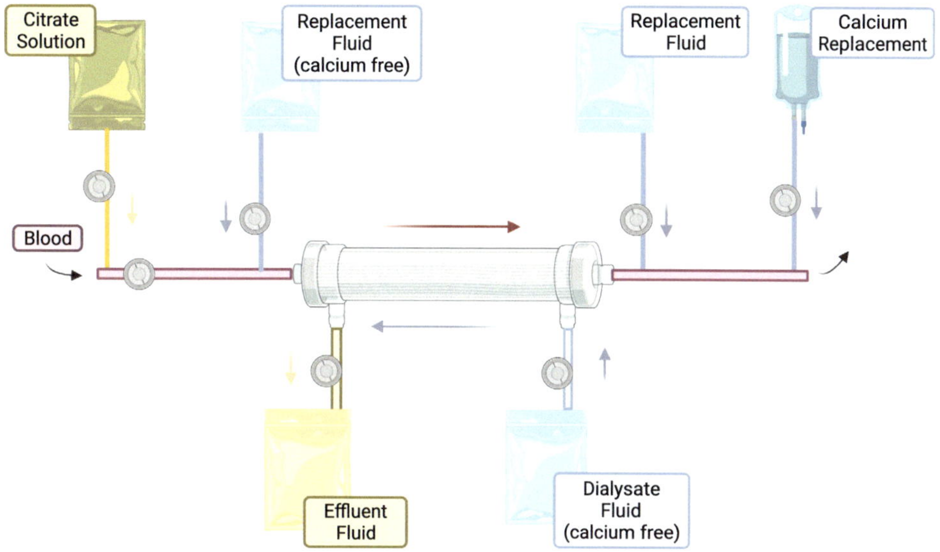


**Figure 4.**
*CVVHDF with regional citrate anticoagulation (RCA). 1) blood, citrate solution, and optional calcium-free replacement fluid mix pre-filter. 2) citrate chelates circulating calcium (required for intrinsic and common pathways of coagulation). 3) calcium-free dialysate (avoiding calcium diffusion from dialysate to blood compartment) circulates countercurrent. 4) replacement fluid and calcium infusion to normalize calcemia are reinjected post-filter.*

(51.2% vs. 53.6%, p = 0.38), fewer bleeding complications (5.1% vs. 16.9%, p < 0.001), but more infections (68% vs. 55.4%, p = 0.002) in RCA compared to systemic heparin [50].

Thorough protocols and expertise in preventing/monitoring complications are required during RCA. The most immediate risk being unreplaced calcium since most complex (Ca-Citrate) is removed by the filter and may lead to severe hypocalcemia. So, one must be extremely careful if the calcium replacement IV line is assembled independently (e.g., CRRT machine continues, but calcium IV line is no longer potent). Citrate metabolism is the next consideration. The liver metabolizes one citrate into three bicarbonates. Even though low bicarbonate replacement and/or dialysate fluids are usually used, RCA is associated with more metabolic alkalosis than heparin [50]. If the liver cannot metabolize citrate, accumulation can be seen and translate in an anion gap metabolic acidosis associated with rise in total calcium levels, but decline ionized calcium. Thus, monitoring total calcium/ionized calcium ratio is helpful and a ratio > 2.5 is a sign of citrate accumulation which is also associated with hypernatremia and hypomagnesemia. Of note, once believed an absolute contraindication of RCA, it has been used safely in patients with liver diseases. A 2019 meta-analysis of 10 observational studies (1241 patients with liver dysfunction) showed no difference in pH, bicarbonate, metabolic alkalosis, lactate levels and total/ionized calcium ratios compared to patients without liver disease [51]. However, a more careful approach than in usual patients should be taken (e.g., tighter biochemical monitoring, lower citrate dose or lower total calcium/ionized calcium threshold) to regularly reassess its safety.

In summary, sustained circuit patency is required to optimize RRT. Understanding filtration fraction is of great help, mainly if anticoagulation is contraindicated. Otherwise, if no other indication mandates systemic anticoagulation, LMWH is the usual first choice for intermittent therapies and RCA for CRRT.

### 3.5 Stopping RRT

Literature is lacking to guide discontinuation of RRT initiated in context of AKI as revealed by the KDIGO-AKI recommendation that simply states "when it is no longer required, because kidney function has recovered to meet patient need or because RRT is no longer consistent with goals of care" [19]. Assessment of recovering kidney function in particularly difficult during RRT. While on intermittent therapy, steady state is not attained therefore excluding use of routine clearance measurements. Interdialytic evaluation of urine volume and creatinine, absolute rise of serum biomarkers (creatinine and BUN), but most probably the rising kinetic over time are frequently used. In a prospective observational study, spontaneous urine output was the best predictor of weaning RRT [52]. A recent systematic review found that urine output prior to RRT discontinuation was the most studied variable, but no threshold value could be determined due to heterogeneity of studies [53]. Pooled analysis found a sensitivity of 66% and specificity of 74% to predict RRT discontinuation, but cut-off values varied from 100 mL increase/day to >1720 mL/24 h. Of note, in one RCT, diuretic-induced diuresis had no benefit on repeated need for RRT or renal recovery [54]. In a retrospective study, a 24-hr urine creatinine clearance >15 ml/min was associated with absence of CRRT need at 14 days [55]. In another study, a 24 h urine creatinine of ≥5.2 mmol on day 2 post-RRT had a 86% sensitivity and 81% specificity of not requiring additional RRT treatment [56]. On the other hand, longer duration of RRT, more severe disease (SOFA score) and older age were associated with restarting RRT which correlated with higher mortality [57].

In summary, clear guidance in stopping RRT is lacking and implies at first a minimal diuresis to avoid marked net fluid accumulation. Then, careful monitoring of clinical (weight, volume balance, diuresis) and paraclinical (serum biomarkers, urine creatinine clearance) data are valuable tools.

## 4. Miscellaneous pearls

Most of the content discussed in previous sections refers to general considerations for understanding and prescribing competently RRT in ICU. However, some challenging situations encountered in clinical practice and pragmatic concerns will be briefly reviewed.

### 4.1 Severe dysnatremias

Mild to moderate dysnatremias are frequent in critically ill patients, especially at initial presentation. Maximum correction rate and approach to treatment differ between guidelines [58]. Though, consensus exists that inadequate correction of chronic severe hyponatremias (<125 mmol/L for >48 hours) should be avoided due to risk of developing osmotic demyelination syndrome (ODS) [59]. Concurrent urgent need for RRT and this condition can be particularly challenging. Since most IHD machines have a minimum sodium of 130 mmol/L, even by prescribing short duration, low blood and dialysate flow rates, overcorrection is a possibility. In the opposite, CRRT has been used effectively at correcting hyponatremias in a predictable manner either by adding a 5% dextrose pre-filter infusion or via customized hypoosmolar dialysate fluids [60].

Limited evidence exists about hypernatremia. Most IHD machines have maximum sodium of 160 mmol/L and CRRT correction protocol has also been published.

Published protocols for **hyponatremias**:

- Rosner and Connor [61] – PMID: 29463598, DOI: 10.2215/CJN.13281117
- Yessayan, Yee [62] – PMID: 2479235, DOI: 10.1053/j.ajkd.2014.01.451

Published protocols for **hypernatremias**:

- Paquette, Goupil [63] – PMID: 27478592, DOI: 10.1093/ckj/sfw036

### 4.2 Acute hepatic failure or acute severe neurologic injury

Patients suffering from acute liver failure (ALF) and acute severe neurologic injury are associated with cerebral edema and increased intracranial pressure. Rapid clearance of plasma solutes/toxins, as in intermittent therapy, can also lead to intracranial pressure (probably by water shift from sudden plasma hypoosmolality) [64].

In ALF, both the KDIGO-AKI and European Associated for Study of Liver (EASL) guidelines recommend CRRT instead of IHD in patients with ALF [19, 65]. Furthermore, RRT may be initiated before usual thresholds since it has been associated with increased transplantation-free survival, probably by clearance of ammonia as hyperammonemia is associated with increased intracranial pressure [66, 67]. Some published protocols used very high doses of CVVHDF (effluent 90 mL/kg/h) [68]. Also, targeting mild hypernatremias (145–150 mmol/L) is recommended in high-risk patients (acute renal failure, ammonia >150 μmol/L, grade IV encephalopathy and use of vasopressor) [65]. Options are customized reinjection and dialysis fluids as discussed above or by adding hypertonic saline perfusion.

### 4.3 Vascular access

Vascular access should deliver stable and sufficient blood flow. In acute care setting, temporary dual-lumen central venous access is used for most patients. Ultrasound-guided catheter insertion is associated with higher successful placement, reduced attempts and time of procedure with less complications [69]. Choosing the site might have short-, mid- and long-term consequences.

Higher rates of catheter dysfunction are observed with femoral and left jugular site compared to right jugular, but no significant difference of urea reduction ratio or RRT downtime was observed [70]. More pneumothoraxes are observed with subclavian access [71].

Risks of catheter-related bloodstream infections and symptomatic deep-vein thrombosis are higher in femoral than subclavian and similar between jugular and femoral [71].

In patient with considerable risk of RRT dependence (mainly with pre-existing advanced CKD), large-bore venous subclavian catheter should be avoided since it can compromise future ipsilateral vascular access due to stenosis.

### 4.4 Disequilibrium syndrome

Dialysis disequilibrium syndrome is a rare, potentially fatal but usually preventable complication of RRT. The pathophysiology is still debated but commonly reports an intracranial osmotic gradient due the rapid removal of urea and osmotic solute by RRT, leading to cerebral edema [72]. The large variation of symptoms and severity, from mild nausea to fatal cerebral herniation makes the diagnosis challenging. The syndrome is mostly reported in ESRD patients with advanced uremia who are initially started on high efficiency/ standard IHD prescription. Patients with ESRD (or with unknown kidney failure duration) should be treated with an adapted low-efficiency IHD prescription, for the first treatments, in order to minimize osmotic shift and risk of disequilibrium syndrome. A progressive increase in dialysate and blood flows and duration can therefore be implemented for the following treatments. Occurrence of this syndrome has also been reported in frail patients with septic shock and AKI even after repeated IHD sessions [73]. In patients who develop symptoms compatible to a disequilibrium syndrome during or quickly after an IHD session, management should include rapid treatment cessation and the administration of osmotic agents (mannitol, hypertonic saline) to quickly raise osmolality, despite the paucity of evidence. However, prevention should still be privileged. The overall risk of dialysis disequilibrium syndrome is lower with PIRRT, and notably reduced in patients treated with CRRT with standard dosing.

### 4.5 Managing IHD hypotension

Intradialytic hypotension is a common complication and can cause further ischemic injury to the recovering kidneys, thereby reducing the probability of renal recovery. Obligate intake in critically ill patients can be high due to nutritional needs and intravenous fluids, which leads to large net UF especially if IHD is performed thrice weekly [74].

| | |
|---|---|
| Minimizing UF | • Avoidance of excessive inter-dialytic weight gain<br>  o Concentrated format of IV drugs<br>  o Reduce enteral free water<br>  o Reduce IV fluid<br>  o Optimize residual urine output with diuretics |
| Dialysis prescription | • Increase the session duration (to reduce the net UF per hour)<br>• Increase the frequency to 4 or 5 IHD sessions per week<br>• Optimize cardioactive electrolytes<br>  o Increase calcium dialysate concentration<br>  o Increase magnesium dialysate concentration<br>• Minimize osmolarity shift during IHD:<br>  o Sodium modeling (gradual increase in sodium dialysate during treatment—may be associated with net sodium gain)<br>• UF modeling (e.g., 50% of total UF during the first third of treatment time, then 50% over the last two-third)<br>• Continuously adapt the UF rate to the residual blood volume<br>• Cooling dialysate (may generate peripherical vasoconstriction and increase the MAP) |
| Pharmacologic interventions | • IV bolus of mannitol (rarely used)<br>• IV bolus of hypertonic albumin<br>• IV vasopressor (preemptive)<br>• Oral midodrine (before or during treatment)<br>• Adjust the timing of antihypertensive and/or antiarrhythmic medications and IHD treatment |

**Table 8.**
*Interventions to minimize intradialytic hypotension.*

While patients in shock or with significant instability should be treated with PIRRT or CRRT (according to local availability), various interventions are associated with reduced risk of intradialytic hypotension during IHD (see **Table 8**). For most of them, despite being widely used in clinical practice, there is still a low level of evidence in context of AKI, as most evidence come from the ESRD population.

## 5. Conclusions

Renal replacement therapies delivered in ICUs are based on one or a combination of the same three basic principles of all extracorporeal blood-based treatments: diffusion, ultrafiltration and convection. Extensive literature has been published to guide clinicians for timing initiation, modality choice and dosing that could be summarized as:

- Timing: For most cases, a conservative approach of watchful waiting is recommended. Accelerated strategies have been associated with added resources, higher infections and RRT dependence without substantial benefits.

- Modality: Neither intermittent vs. continuous nor diffusion vs. convection have shown clear superiority. Hence, pragmatical considerations and mostly local expertise guide selection.

- Dosing: For intermittent therapy, ensuring volume balance, metabolic homeostasis and a delivered $Kt/V \geq 1.2$/session or $URR \geq 67\%$ seems adequate. For CRRT, prescribing an effluent volume of 25–30 mL/kg/h to ensure a 20-25 mL/kg/h delivered is recommended in most scenarios.

Significant differences are observed between guidelines and clinical practice regarding anticoagulation and timing of initiation. Forthcoming guidelines updates will further help to standardize approach in RRT prescription. However, data are scarce to guide termination of RRT; large prospective trials are needed before strong recommendations could be made. Finally, usual prescriptions could not be adequate for some patients with challenging scenarios, where an individualized strategies need to be applied.

## Acknowledgements

All figures have been created by the authors using BioRender.com. IntechOpen Ltd. can use and share these figures without additional permission.

## Conflict of interest

The authors declare no conflict of interest.

## Author details

Dominic Godbout[1], Philippe Lachance[2] and Jean-Maxime Côté[3]*

1 Quebec Heart and Lung Institute, Quebec, Canada

2 University of Quebec Health Centre, Quebec, Canada

3 University of Montreal Health Centre, Montreal, Canada

*Address all correspondence to: jean-maxime.cote@umontreal.ca

## References

[1] Mehta RL et al.. Spectrum of acute renal failure in the intensive care unit: The PICARD experience. Kidney International. 2004;**66**(4):1613-1621

[2] Hoste EA et al.. Epidemiology of acute kidney injury in critically ill patients: The multinational AKI-EPI study. Intensive Care Medicine. 2015; **41**(8):1411-1423

[3] Hsu RK et al.. Temporal changes in incidence of dialysis-requiring AKI. J Am Soc Nephrol. 2013;**24**(1):37-42

[4] Featherstone PJ, Ball CM. A brief history of haemodialysis and continuous renal replacement therapy. Anaesthesia and Intensive Care. 2019;**47**(3):220-222

[5] Claure-Del Granado R, Clark WR. Continuous renal replacement therapy principles. Seminars in Dialysis. 2021; **34**(6):398-405

[6] Basile C, Davenport A, Blankestijn PJ. Why choose high volume online post-dilution hemodiafiltration? Journal of Nephrology. 2017;**30**(2):181-186

[7] Hellman T, Uusalo P, Jarvisalo MJ. Renal replacement techniques in septic shock. International Journal of Molecular Sciences. 2021;**22**(19)

[8] Cote JM et al.. Intermittent convective therapies in patients with acute kidney injury: A systematic review with meta-analysis. Blood Purification. 2022;**51**(1):75-86

[9] Tandukar S, Palevsky PM. Continuous renal replacement therapy: Who, when, why, and how. Chest. 2019; **155**(3):626-638

[10] Section 2: AKI definition. Kidney Int Suppl (2011). 2012;**2**(1):19-36

[11] Venkataraman R, Kellum JA. Defining acute renal failure: The RIFLE criteria. Journal of Intensive Care Medicine. 2007;**22**(4):187-193

[12] Zarbock A et al.. Effect of early vs delayed initiation of renal replacement therapy on mortality in critically ill patients with acute kidney injury: The ELAIN randomized clinical trial. JAMA. 2016;**315**(20):2190-2199

[13] Gaudry S et al. Initiation strategies for renal-replacement therapy in the intensive care unit. The New England Journal of Medicine. 2016;**375**(2):122-133

[14] Barbar SD et al. Timing of renal-replacement therapy in patients with acute kidney injury and sepsis. The New England Journal of Medicine. 2018; **379**(15):1431-1442

[15] Investigators S-A et al. Timing of initiation of renal-replacement therapy in acute kidney injury. The New England Journal of Medicine. 2020;**383**(3): 240-251

[16] Klein SJ et al. Biomarkers for prediction of renal replacement therapy in acute kidney injury: A systematic review and meta-analysis. Intensive Care Medicine. 2018;**44**(3):323-336

[17] Chen JJ et al. Furosemide stress test as a predictive marker of acute kidney injury progression or renal replacement therapy: A systemic review and meta-analysis. Critical Care. 2020; **24**(1):202

[18] Ostermann M et al. Recommendations on acute kidney injury biomarkers from the acute disease quality initiative consensus conference: A consensus statement. JAMA Network Open. 2020;**3**(10):e2019209

[19] Khwaja A. KDIGO clinical practice guidelines for acute kidney injury. Nephron. Clinical Practice. 2012;**120**(4): c179-c184

[20] Mehta RL et al. A randomized clinical trial of continuous versus intermittent dialysis for acute renal failure. Kidney International. 2001; **60**(3):1154-1163

[21] Guerin C et al. Intermittent versus continuous renal replacement therapy for acute renal failure in intensive care units: Results from a multicenter prospective epidemiological survey. Intensive Care Medicine. 2002;**28**(10): 1411-1418

[22] Gasparovic V et al. Continuous renal replacement therapy (CRRT) or intermittent hemodialysis (IHD)–what is the procedure of choice in critically ill patients? Renal Failure. 2003;**25**(5): 855-862

[23] Augustine JJ et al. A randomized controlled trial comparing intermittent with continuous dialysis in patients with ARF. American Journal of Kidney Diseases. 2004;**44**(6):1000-1007

[24] Vinsonneau C et al. Continuous venovenous haemodiafiltration versus intermittent haemodialysis for acute renal failure in patients with multiple-organ dysfunction syndrome: A multicentre randomised trial. Lancet. 2006;**368**(9533):379-385

[25] Lins RL et al. Intermittent versus continuous renal replacement therapy for acute kidney injury patients admitted to the intensive care unit: Results of a randomized clinical trial. Nephrology, Dialysis, Transplantation. 2009;**24**(2): 512-518

[26] Schefold JC et al. The effect of continuous versus intermittent renal replacement therapy on the outcome of critically ill patients with acute renal failure (CONVINT): A prospective randomized controlled trial. Critical Care. 2014;**18**(1):R11

[27] Peters SA et al. Haemodiafiltration and mortality in end-stage kidney disease patients: A pooled individual participant data analysis from four randomized controlled trials. Nephrology, Dialysis, Transplantation. 2016;**31**(6):978-984

[28] Friedrich JO et al. Hemofiltration compared to hemodialysis for acute kidney injury: Systematic review and meta-analysis. Critical Care. 2012;**16**(4):R146

[29] Sigwalt F et al. Clinical complications of continuous renal replacement therapy. Contributions to Nephrology. 2018;**194**:109-117

[30] Palevsky PM et al. KDOQI US commentary on the 2012 KDIGO clinical practice guideline for acute kidney injury. American Journal of Kidney Diseases. 2013;**61**(5):649-672

[31] Lowrie E, Lew N. The urea reduction ratio (URR). A simple method for evaluating hemodialysis treatment. 1992

[32] Daugirdas JT, Depner TA. A nomogram approach to hemodialysis urea modeling. American Journal of Kidney Diseases. 1994;**23**(1):33-40

[33] Jorres A et al. A European renal best practice (ERBP) position statement on the kidney disease improving global outcomes (KDIGO) clinical practice guidelines on acute kidney injury: Part 2: Renal replacement therapy. Nephrology, Dialysis, Transplantation. 2013;**28**(12): 2940-2945

[34] Network VNARFT et al. Intensity of renal support in critically ill patients

with acute kidney injury. The New England Journal of Medicine. 2008; **359**(1):7-20

[35] Ronco C et al. Effects of different doses in continuous veno-venous haemofiltration on outcomes of acute renal failure: A prospective randomised trial. Lancet. 2000;**356**(9223):26-30

[36] Bouman CSC et al. Effects of early high-volume continuous venovenous hemofiltration on survival and recovery of renal function in intensive care patients with acute renal failure: A prospective, randomized trial. Critical Care Medicine. 2002;**30**(10):2205-2211

[37] Saudan P et al. Adding a dialysis dose to continuous hemofiltration increases survival in patients with acute renal failure. Kidney International. 2006; **70**(7):1312-1317

[38] Tolwani AJ et al. Standard versus high-dose CVVHDF for ICU-related acute renal failure. J Am Soc Nephrol. 2008;**19**(6):1233-1238

[39] Investigators RRTS et al. Intensity of continuous renal-replacement therapy in critically ill patients. The New England Journal of Medicine. 2009;**361**(17): 1627-1638

[40] Schetz M. Anticoagulation in continuous renal replacement therapy. Contributions to Nephrology. 2001;**132**: 283-303

[41] Joannidis M, Oudemans-van Straaten HM. Clinical review: Patency of the circuit in continuous renal replacement therapy. Critical Care. 2007;**11**(4):218

[42] Fischer KG. Essentials of anticoagulation in hemodialysis. Hemodialysis International. 2007;**11**(2): 178-189

[43] O'Shea SI, Ortel TL, Kovalik EC. Alternative methods of anticoagulation for dialysis-dependent patients with heparin-induced thrombocytopenia. Seminars in Dialysis. 2003;**16**(1):61-67

[44] Kalpatthi R, Kiss JE. Thrombotic thrombocytopenic purpura, heparin-induced thrombocytopenia, and disseminated intravascular coagulation. Critical Care Clinics. 2020;**36**(2):357-377

[45] Lim W, Cook DJ, Crowther MA. Safety and efficacy of low molecular weight heparins for hemodialysis in patients with end-stage renal failure: A meta-analysis of randomized trials. J Am Soc Nephrol. 2004;**15**(12):3192-3206

[46] Joannidis M et al. Enoxaparin vs. unfractionated heparin for anticoagulation during continuous veno-venous hemofiltration: A randomized controlled crossover study. Intensive Care Medicine. 2007;**33**(9):1571-1579

[47] Goet E, Wentz B, Frank RD. Regional citrate anticoagulation protocol suitable for intermittent hemodialysis and post-dilution hemodiafiltration. Clinical Nephrology. 2021;**96**(2):90-95

[48] Kindgen-Milles D, Brandenburger T, Dimski T. Regional citrate anticoagulation for continuous renal replacement therapy. Current Opinion in Critical Care. 2018;**24**(6):450-454

[49] Bai M et al. Citrate versus heparin anticoagulation for continuous renal replacement therapy: An updated meta-analysis of RCTs. Intensive Care Medicine. 2015;**41**(12):2098-2110

[50] Zarbock A et al. Effect of regional citrate anticoagulation vs systemic heparin anticoagulation during continuous kidney replacement therapy on dialysis filter life span and mortality among critically ill patients with acute

kidney injury: A randomized clinical trial. JAMA. 2020;**324**(16):1629-1639

[51] Zhang W et al. Safety and efficacy of regional citrate anticoagulation for continuous renal replacement therapy in liver failure patients: A systematic review and meta-analysis. Critical Care. 2019;**23**(1):22

[52] Uchino S et al. Discontinuation of continuous renal replacement therapy: A post hoc analysis of a prospective multicenter observational study. Critical Care Medicine. 2009;**37**(9):2576-2582

[53] Katulka RJ et al. Determining the optimal time for liberation from renal replacement therapy in critically ill patients: A systematic review and meta-analysis (DOnE RRT). Critical Care. 2020;**24**(1):50

[54] van der Voort PH et al. Furosemide does not improve renal recovery after hemofiltration for acute renal failure in critically ill patients: A double blind randomized controlled trial. Critical Care Medicine. 2009;**37**(2):533-538

[55] Shealy C, Campbell R, Hey J. 24-hr creatinine clearance as a guide for CRRT withdrawal: A retrospective study (abstr). Blood Purification. 2003; **21**:192

[56] Viallet N et al. Daily urinary creatinine predicts the weaning of renal replacement therapy in ICU acute kidney injury patients. Annals of Intensive Care. 2016;**6**(1):71

[57] Wu VC et al. Risk factors of early redialysis after weaning from postoperative acute renal replacement therapy. Intensive Care Medicine. 2008; **34**(1):101-108

[58] Hoorn EJ, Zietse R. Diagnosis and treatment of hyponatremia: Compilation of the guidelines. J Am Soc Nephrol. 2017;**28**(5):1340-1349

[59] Sterns RH, Riggs JE, Schochet SS Jr. Osmotic demyelination syndrome following correction of hyponatremia. The New England Journal of Medicine. 1986;**314**(24):1535-1542

[60] Tandukar S et al. Severe hyponatremia and continuous renal replacement therapy: Safety and effectiveness of low-sodium dialysate. Kidney Med. 2020;**2**(4): 437-449

[61] Rosner MH, Connor MJ Jr. Management of Severe Hyponatremia with continuous renal replacement therapies. Clinical Journal of the American Society of Nephrology. 2018; **13**(5):787-789

[62] Yessayan L et al. Treatment of severe hyponatremia in patients with kidney failure: Role of continuous venovenous hemofiltration with low-sodium replacement fluid. American Journal of Kidney Diseases. 2014;**64**(2):305-310

[63] Paquette F et al. Continuous venovenous hemofiltration using customized replacement fluid for acute kidney injury with severe hypernatremia. Clinical Kidney Journal. 2016;**9**(4):540-542

[64] Lin CM et al. Intracranial pressure fluctuation during hemodialysis in renal failure patients with intracranial hemorrhage. Acta Neurochirurgica. Supplement. 2008;**101**:141-144

[65] European Association for the Study of the Liver. Electronic address, e.e.e et al. EASL clinical practical guidelines on the management of acute (fulminant) liver failure. Journal of Hepatology. 2017;**66**(5): 1047-1081

[66] Warrillow S et al. Continuous renal replacement therapy and its impact on hyperammonaemia in acute liver failure. Critical Care and Resuscitation. 2020; **22**(2):158-165

[67] Cardoso FS et al. Continuous renal replacement therapy is associated with reduced serum ammonia levels and mortality in acute liver failure. Hepatology. 2018;**67**(2):711-720

[68] Slack AJ et al. Ammonia clearance with haemofiltration in adults with liver disease. Liver International. 2014;**34**(1): 42-48

[69] Rabindranath KS et al. Use of real-time ultrasound guidance for the placement of hemodialysis catheters: A systematic review and meta-analysis of randomized controlled trials. American Journal of Kidney Diseases. 2011;**58**(6): 964-970

[70] Parienti JJ et al. Catheter dysfunction and dialysis performance according to vascular access among 736 critically ill adults requiring renal replacement therapy: A randomized controlled study. Critical Care Medicine. 2010;**38**(4): 1118-1125

[71] Parienti JJ et al. Intravascular complications of central venous catheterization by insertion site. The New England Journal of Medicine. 2015; **373**(13):1220-1229

[72] Arieff AI. Dialysis disequilibrium syndrome: Current concepts on pathogenesis and prevention. Kidney International. 1994;**45**(3): 629-635

[73] Shaikh N, Louon A, Hanssens Y. Fatal dialysis disequilibrium syndrome: A tale of two patients. Journal of Emergencies, Trauma, and Shock. 2010; **3**(3):300

[74] Sharma S, Waikar SS. Intradialytic hypotension in acute kidney injury requiring renal replacement therapy. Seminars in Dialysis. 2017;**30**(6):553-558

Chapter 4

# Trauma Resuscitation, Mass Casualty Incident Management and COVID 19: Experience from a South African Trauma Unit

*Naadiyah Laher*


## Abstract

The COVID 19 pandemic has spanned 2 years and is still ongoing with many questions arising. We attempt to answer some pertinent questions with literature as well as anecdotal evidence from our facility. To describe any changes to the resuscitation of trauma patients during the COVID 19 pandemic if any. During the COVID 19 pandemic, Johannesburg a city in the Gauteng Province of South Africa experienced civil unrest and a fire at one of its trauma units, this resulted in a mass casualty incident (MCI) at the only functional trauma unit in the public sector. Results of this observational study will be elucidated. Focus is placed on PPE protocols, trauma resuscitations, MCI management, triage principles and the changing surgeon's role within the pandemic.


**Keywords:** trauma resuscitation, mass casualty incident (MCI), PPE, triage, COVID

## 1. Introduction

The COVID 19 pandemic has spanned 2 years and is still ongoing, this pandemic has had significant impact on all healthcare professionals. The spectrum of its effect is vast ranging from PPE protocols for infectious diseases, training of healthcare professionals, research, burn out and the response to a never- ending global mass casualty incident (MCI). Reviewing the literature brings about many questions, some of which are answered by anecdotal evidence within our setting and some that have been published. The literature in the past 2 years with regards to covid and its effect in different settings is extensive and ever changing. We attempt to answer some pertinent questions with literature as well as anecdotal evidence from our facility. Focus is placed on PPE protocols, trauma resuscitations, MCI management, triage principles and the changing surgeon's role within the pandemic.

## 2. PPE and trauma

PPE has been an integral part of the ATLS principles of a trauma resuscitation and has been taught globally [1]. With the advent of the Covid 19 pandemic, more focus has been placed on PPE protocols for not only resuscitation but for all patient interaction due to the infectious nature of the virus and the unknown state of the patient at first interaction. These PPE protocols have evolved over the last 2 years with the ongoing research into the spread of COVID 19 and all its variants from full PPE and fomite transmission to no fomite transmission and basic PPE such as a plastic apron, visor and N95 for all patient interaction, whereas the vast public is encouraged with social distancing, hand sanitizing and either surgical or cloth face masks [2, 3]. These evolving protocols have no effect on the trauma resuscitation, as the basis here is healthcare professionals safety from all bodily fluids in a high risk, life threatening situation. **Could this be the reason for a low positivity rate among healthcare professionals in the trauma surgical discipline?** In an attempt to answer this question, I provide you with unpublished data from our facility due to a lack of appropriate literature available to answer this question.

Our facility was faced with a MCI due to civil unrest in the week of 9–16 July 2021. At the same time we were experiencing the 3rd COVID wave, with an adjusted level 4 lockdown, this entailed a curfew from 9 pm to 4 am, and no alcohol sales. Our neighboring hospital (18 km away) with the only other functional trauma unit in our Metropolitan was shut down due to a fire and with the civil unrest, all patients were seen in the only functional trauma facility. Although the numbers of patients and procedures done increased, patient positivity rate was 9% below the national average of 29.1% at the time [4]. Only two doctors of a total of forty tested positive during this time (5%). This was with the adherence to standard PPE protocols according to ATLS principles with the inclusion of a N95 masks (unpublished data).

Similarly In Nigeria full PPE was used when intubating patients, and when performing an emergency room thoracotomy while standard precautions were used for ICD insertions [5]. Globally we have seen many doctors and healthcare professionals testing positive for covid and in the infancy of the pandemic, many had succumbed to the virus. Most of which were involved in patient care of COVID positive patients with the adherence of PPE protocols [6]. **Again, one would question why this is the case? Is it due to the combination of the burden of COVID positive patients seen by the individual and the burn out experienced by many which ultimately weaken the immune system?** A meta-analysis done in 2021 has failed to answer this question [6]. However the changing PPE protocols and COVID infections of healthcare personnel, community acquired or nosocomial, did not change how we would resuscitate a trauma patient with an unknown covid status, we adhered to basic principles, which was guided by ATLS principles [1].

## 3. Trauma resuscitation, patient management and covid

One cannot comment on a trauma resuscitation without mentioning the ATLS resuscitation principles [1]. As part of any trauma resuscitation, there are many life- saving procedure that need to be done with urgency under aseptic techniques, as a result trauma resus bays are well stocked with all the equipment within arm's reach [1]. Due to the concern for fomite transmission, some trauma departments changed the layout of their resuscitation area and removing equipment to a different area that is remote from the patient interaction [7]. Livingstone et al. removed all equipment from their trauma resuscitation bays. They designated hot, warm, and cold zones around the patient, where a hot zone involved direct patient contact, a cold zone was a significant distance from patient interaction, where equipment was kept, and the warm zone was the zone in between hot and cold where equipment was transferred on a table. This was in keeping with the EPA guidelines [7]. Logistically, this would hamper an efficient resuscitation and it can now be seen that it was not necessary due to the lack of fomite transmission [3].

In an effort to conserve PPE, only the staff in the hot zone donned and doffed full PPE, in our setting we also experienced a shortage of PPE and therefore one gown with an N95 and a visor was issued per shift to each healthcare practitioner (shifts lasted either 12 or 24 hours) [7]. However, this can be adapted to the ever-changing PPE protocols [2].

I would like to bring your attention back to our MCI with the low positivity rates. We have a 15- bay resuscitation area with each bay having its own monitors and life- saving equipment. We did not change our resus area at all and again we had low positivity rates (unpublished data). This adds to the evidence for non- fomite transmission [3].

The first focus of the ATLS resuscitation is airway management with its inherent risk for transmission during intubation as an aerosolizing generating event [8]. At the beginning of the pandemic, the use of intubating boxes was advocated. However practically they were not feasible and seemed to hamper airway management [9]. What worked well for us was a video laryngoscope, equipment that was previously not available in our trauma resuscitation area and was reserved for the use by anesthetists [10]. This has also been substantiated in the literature with a meta-analysis [11]. Thus the pandemic benefitted us in that we could hone in on this new skill and gain confidence in the use of it.

COVID positivity or screening never became part of our trauma resuscitation protocols. All patients were treated as PUIs (patients under investigation) meaning their covid status was unknown and all patients that were admitted or required a surgical procedure were tested. If the status of the patient was unknown, they were again operated on a PUIs. We had no dedicated PUIs theater as most acute care surgical and trauma patients were operated on with their covid results being unknown. This was largely due to PCR results turnaround time of about 12 hours if tested after 4 pm and 2 hours if before 4 pm. Surgeons used disposable gowns (a change in the usual theater attire), visors, and masks, which were a N95 instead of a surgical mask. Anesthetic staff occasionally used half-face elastomeric respirator with P100 filters if they were intubating the patient, of note, these were not supplied by the hospital but instead purchased on the own accord of the anesthetist.

Post operatively patients went to the ward which was also a PUI area and only once covid status was known would they be transferred to the covid wards or ICU if a positive result was found. The main nine bed Trauma ICU required a COVID negative result before admission of the patient and therefore a patient would be housed within the ward ventilated and ongoing resus was continued until a result was known and the patient was accepted for admission to the Trauma ICU.

Again, I would like to mention that although our ward was considered a PUI ward, as well as a COVID negative ward as only the COVID positive patients would be moved out once their result was known. We still only had a 9% positivity rate within the unit during our MCI (unpublished data).

In Nigeria, their trauma protocols were adjusted. Patients were screened in their triage area for fever and flu like symptoms not related to their traumatic injury, contact and travel history. Suspected cases were moved to a designated area to be seen by the hospital COVID 19 team (review and testing) while the trauma team continued the resus. Suspected patients were given a surgical mask [5]. This change in protocols places more emphasis on COVID instead of the traumatic injury. Due to social distancing their resus area capacity decreased from twelve beds to eight beds. The most senior person managed the airway in full PPE. With regards to surgical procedures an N95 and face shield was added to their PPE protocol in theater and the most experienced personnel operated to decrease operative time, hampering training [5]. They again focused on COVID by adding signs and symptoms of covid and travel history to the AMPLE history changing the acronym to SAMPLET. Surgical protocols were also changed, with the focus shifting to COVID, if a patient was covid positive, non-operative or delayed repairs were encouraged [5]. These decisions should be based on the patient's trauma burden and physiology. We made neither of these changes to our protocols, our focus remained on trauma, the only difference covid made was changing the location of the patient. However, we need to do a formal audit to quantify if our covid positive patients' outcomes were significantly different to their covid negative counterparts. In some areas the trauma burden has decreased with the increase of covid thereby providing us with an ongoing MCI and an approach to this needs to be defined [12].

## 4. Mass casualty incidents (MCIs)

MCIs are defined as events where the number of patients exceed the local resources (human or equipment). These events can occur remotely to the health facility or within the health facility. All the literature on mass casualties come from the trauma surgical discipline [13]. The questions we now need to ask is, **combined with COVID, do trauma protocols and triage principles need to change? Is there more that we can learn from this?** In an attempt to answer these questions, we revert to the literature. One must be cognizant of the fact that with the covid pandemic all patients essentially have a breathing problem, if one must consider ATLS principles, some of which may require invasive ventilation [1].

Tankel and Einov defined specific objectives that need to be planned for in a MCI, namely equipment and consumables, transport, hospital capacity, training, education, and debriefing, command and control and communication [13]. These are the same principles in disaster management, some of which will be highlighted in this text. These concepts are echoed by the WHO guidelines which involves a multisectoral planning which include national governments and healthcare personnel, starting at facility level to international level [14].

Data from the US stems from terrorism attacks and mass shooting events and have influenced MCI protocols [13]. The major difference between a MCI in a trauma setting and a pandemic is the length of the mass casualty. Most MCIs last 24–48 hours and thereafter there is a return to normal duties, which allows for a period of debriefing. But this MCI has lasted 2 years and there has been no return to 'normalcy' [15]. **So, can we truly extrapolate from MCI in the trauma setting to a pandemic? When do we return to pre pandemic triage/MCI principles when the MCI is prolonged?**

Planning ahead, stock piling of equipment and consumables are integral to a response to a MCI [13, 14]. However, consumables are a limiting factor in MCIs as well as in a pandemic as evidenced by the global oxygen supply shortage and ventilator shortage [16]. Tankel and Einov suggest that regional instead of local (individual hospital) stock piling is more cost effective, however maintenance of the consumables is questionable and therefore may not be functional when needed. One also needs to define MCI specific equipment for example during the pandemic this translated to oxygen and ventilators but in a trauma, setting could be theater capacity, availability of trauma surgeons and blood and blood products [13].

### 4.1 What happens when the supply of global resources outweighs the demand be it oxygen or human resources?

Our healthcare professionals have lost their lives from being on the frontline and burn out has become more evident than before [6, 17]. Training of new healthcare professionals have also been hampered in the past 2 years of the pandemic because all they now know is how to manage a COVID patient. Airway skills have become a selective skill reserved for anesthetist and the most senior personnel at the expense of the junior doctors that have started out [5, 8].

To confound matters while experiencing the COVID pandemic we needed to deal with a disaster (mass evacuation of a hospital due to a fire), this resulted in the hospital closure and the majority of patients being redirected to our facility. This was even further confounded by enduring a MCI when civil unrest led to a flood of patients in our trauma unit.

The evacuation of a hospital due to a fire was largely driven by healthcare professionals selflessly moving patients (immobile patients, in their beds) to evacuations points in smoke covered corridors with no oxygen supplies while emergency fire personnel battled the blaze. The loss of a health facility compounded the effects of a pandemic on the loco regional facilities.

With this said the loco regional functional hospitals can change their triage processes and therefore certain hospitals can only accept P1 and other hospitals can accept P2 and P3 patients thereby distributing the load [13]. Prehospital services and healthcare facilities (receiving and disaster area) should have effective communication for this to be feasible, disaster committees should be established in the sending and receiving facilities. Efficient communication is integral to the management of any disaster or MCI [15].

Our facility was on the receiving end of the fire, 150 patients were evacuated to our facility without communication to the team onsite. Both the on- call trauma and acute care surgical units had to manage current acute patients in their respective areas as well as the patients evacuated to their facility. The discrepancy here was that a disaster team should have been established at the receiving hospital to manage evacuated patients. This should not have been the responsibility of the on-call trauma and acute care surgical units. Emergency services that transported patients to our facility were also used to transport patients to the relevant wards as we did not have the capacity (porters) available to do this, therefore the need for non-healthcare personnel should also be considered e.g. cleaners, porters etc. [13].

The burden on the facility was significant as bed capacity was reduced due to reallocations for COVID patients. Unique to South Africa is that a large percentage of our population lives below the poverty line in informal settlements, which are quite densely populated, you could have at least ten people living in a 1-bedroom shack (informal dwelling) [18]. Therefore, our patients could not self- isolate at home and a facility was opened for this specific reason NASREC, previously an events area. This was specific for patients not requiring hospital admission and no oxygen requirements. It was purely for patients that were unable to self- isolate safely at home. This was an attempt to lessen the load on secondary and tertiary level institutes.

Going back to the MCI specific to trauma the riots from the civil unrest. This event was not anticipated and therefore could not be planned for especially during a covid pandemic and with the neighboring hospital trauma unit closed due to a fire. We experienced many bottle necks for example CT scanners availability and theater capacity despite more staff being mobilized to respond to the disaster. We were also unable to mobilize staff from outside the hospital as it was not safe to travel to the hospital. Therefore, disaster committees should focus on training, education and debriefing, treatment protocols that are disease or injury specific and should be aim at a level appropriate for all heath care specialist not just trauma surgeons or infectious disease specialists [13, 15].

Due to the sheer burden of P3 patients, we developed a strategy for quick reference as to the patient's condition and progress of management. Labels were placed on patients and were used to indicate injuries, results of investigations and what the patients were awaiting as a quick reference with no need to go locate the patient file. This is planning whilst one is in the midst of a MCI but was successful and will be used for planning of future MCI within our institution. Therefore, a response to a MCI is an ongoing process.

With regards to training over the last 2 years. Interns have mostly been exposed to the management of covid patients which has largely been protocol based. They have missed opportunities related to procedures specifically that of airway management which many have reserved for the most senior staff [5, 10]. In the surgical spectrum, elective procedures have been stopped thus decreasing exposure of surgical trainees. Despite discrepancies in training and being reallocated to manage patients that is not within your field of expertise, burnout has come to the fore [17, 19, 20]. Many healthcare personnel have experienced burnout largely due to the pandemic/mass casualty spanning 2 years currently and leaving no time to debrief or recuperate after each wave [17]. Human resources are a scarce commodity as well as being constraints by a budget for monetary compensation, as seen by healthcare professionals working long hours risking their lives as well as that of the household [15].

Command and control of a mass casualty or disaster must consist of healthcare professionals that are clinically active, to know what is happening on the floor as well as management and politicians and policy makers. These committees should be established locally, regionally, nationally, and even internationally depending on the nature of the MCI [13, 14]. Elective theaters, emergency theaters, ICU, physicians, surgeons, allieds, nursing staff, porters, radiographers, and radiology form integral components of the response team to these events. Special types of patients should also be considered especially those that are time dependent such as cancer patients [13]. Once a SOP (standard operating procedure) was established for the covid response and the relocation of patients due to the fire. Chemotherapy and radiotherapy as well as surgical procedures for patients with malignancies were prioritized. Oncological services such as chemo- and radiotherapy were halted transiently as they were only available at the hospital that was closed due to the fire, however rapid communication with other hospitals and the fast tracking of the establishment of a chemotherapy service at our hospital assisted with this issue. Transport for these patients were also arranged to these facilities, not to impede these patients from receiving oncological services. Communication needs to be bi-directional top down and bottom up, so that protocols are practical and feasible with real-time feedback [13].

Coccolini et al. defined four phases in disaster management namely mitigation, planning, response, and recovery. Mitigation, this is the preemptive planning stage to reduce the effect of MCIs however the protocols of COVID was ever changing (PPE, isolation days, lockdown periods, economics changing policy) and therefore the planning stage is an evolving stage [2, 3, 8]. Planning requires practice of protocols for feasibility however there was no time with the pandemic to practice, it's been an ongoing practice session for the past 2 years as such good communication (local, regional, national, international, NPOs) has become imperative [15]. The response phase entails activation, notification, and initial response. Therefore, the need to identify a state of disaster and activation of the relevant teams, and a central Command structure (local, regional, or national) [15]. The major issues with the covid pandemic and its associated disaster management is the ever-changing protocols resulting in the planning, practice and response phases never ending. You also need buy in from all stake holders, however medical personnel have also become hesitant in accepting these ever-changing protocols. As healthcare providers we have lost the trust of the global population by changing protocols largely due to the lack of understanding of the research process [2, 8, 10, 15]. The final stage is recovery, which entails staff debriefing, however with the many waves of the pandemic we have not reached this phase in 2 years, resulting in burn out and significant strain on the mental health of many healthcare professionals [15, 17]. With these ever-changing protocols of covid and a prolonged MCI, **do we still utilize triage principles as before, or do we adapt them to the current pandemic?**

## 5. Triage principles

The Federal healthcare resilience task force kept the trauma triage principles unchanged, with just the addition of the awareness of COVID 19 and the prehospital use of PPE [21]. This was also the case within our facility. A common theme prehospital and within hospital resus is the decreased number of healthcare personnel involved in the resus and airway management was by the most senior first responder [7, 21]. With specific reference to the covid pandemic and MCIs, crowd control becomes important [21].

It has been stated that during the current pandemic, it is unable to "discern the likelihood of survival of trauma patients relative to the potential for having concomitant COVID 19 is not possible [21]. One would disagree with this statement, there are many trauma scores that relate burden of injury to mortality and therefore concomitant COVID or the suspicion of covid played no role in our triage process. The burden of injury and the survivability of the injury enabled our triage process according to trauma principles.

Supportive and palliative care is an ethical principle that forms part of any MCIs [13, 15]. During this pandemic this has come to the fore due to shortages of ICU beds, ventilators and even Oxygen and the overwhelming demand [16]. Palliative care has become integral to triage during this longstanding MCIs that is the COVID Pandemic [22].

At our facility, most of our trauma patients are young males and were incidental or asymptomatic covid positive results. During the pandemic in a trauma setting, we still focused on the principles of triage according to the trauma burden and was more focused on the survivability of the injuries sustained and not the patients covid status [1]. Their covid status may have complicated their surgical course and lead to unexpected deaths or morbidities but it did not hamper their treatment. If at all, it might have given them resources which would not have been otherwise available. Our unit only has a nine bed Trauma ICU, but with the COVID pandemic a general ward was converted to a thirty seven bed COVID ICU, so if not for their COVID status some patients may not have received the critical care that they needed. We have discussed the covid pandemic with regards to PPE, MCIs and resuscitation, extrapolating principles from surgery, but **what has been the surgeon's role in the pandemic?**

## 6. The surgeon and COVID

Elster et al. commented that surgeons responded by postponing elective surgery, however this was a misnomer. Most electives are time sensitive malignant cases [23]. At our facility we instituted the Covid scoring system (NDOH technical working group on COVID 19) as well as a vetting committee and as a result our oncological procedures and services continued.

With regards to COVID positive elective cases they were postponed to either when the patient was asymptomatic for 72 hours and two negative covid tests 24 hours apart [23]. At our facility we initially postponed to 2 weeks post covid infection and as evidence become available our protocols change to 8 weeks post covid, in keeping with the current literature [24]. No repeat covid tested were requested on patients previously tested positive.

In order to protect staff members from a prolonged MCI Elster et al., implemented a few protocols, namely, Screening of outpatients, testing patients before entering the hospital, limiting OPD and seeing only the medically needed and time sensitive cases, avoiding burnout and unprotected exposure to infected patients, encouraging telemedicine and all meetings to be done virtually [23]. These protocols have also been implemented within our facility except for the avoidance of burn out. Surgeons and interns were mobilized to work in COVID units. Critical care training is included in the curriculum for surgical residents as well as having experience with critical care in the wards due to the shortage of critical care beds within specialized units. These covid duties were in addition to their surgical responsibilities and therefore impossible to avoid burnout. Surgeons have skills that are geared towards dealing with the COVID pandemic, these skills arise from their experiences in MCIs in the combat and trauma setting as well as their critical care experiences [23].

Literature is populated with the surgeon's role in the pandemic [25, 26]. Acute care surgeons assisted by converting post operative recovery areas into ICUs to increase critical care capacity, which were managed by critical care trained surgeons. The less severe covid patients were managed by surgeons with no critical care experience as well as taking on acute care surgical responsibilities of themselves and the critically trained surgeons. Non critically trained surgeons were prepared for their covid responsibilities by undergoing a 1 week catch up course involving antibiotic and ventilatory strategies as well as specific covid protocols. There were times when they were teamed up with physician intensivists or small teams consisting of members from all specialties with one team leader [25, 26]. All electives and research activities were stopped to increase human resources [25]. The strategy of Giogola et al. involved weekly virtual meetings for updates, a tiered approach adapted from the SCCM which resulted in intensivist burn out as it was top heavy [25].

In a London Trauma unit, they anticipated a staff illness rate of 30%, to negate this they allowed high risk personnel to provide off site support virtually or telephonically which translated to a staff illness rate of 10%. Again, surgical responsibilities were decreased by stopping electives and the application of lock downs decreased the trauma burden [26]. OPD were done telephonically or virtually. With the covid pandemic social media played an important role, however there were concerns with patient confidentiality and therefore social media was sanctioned nationally and only allowed within a hospital. These platforms were used to disseminate the latest peer reviewed information but at times humor and outburst were also shared, which can be expected from staff experiencing a prolonged MCI resulting in burnout with no time to debrief [26]. Social media may have assisted with information dissemination within a hospital, but difficulties were seen with communication from a central command to those on the frontline [26].

Due to the re-deployment of anesthetic and surgical staff to covid units, non-operative management was favored, and theaters were transformed to ICUs, impacting training of fellows and residents negatively. To compensate for this deficit, many extended their training time [26]. In our setting surgical management remained according to surgical principles and protocols pre covid and not dictated by the patient's covid status.

To assist with healthcare professional well-being, which was affected by loss job opportunities, uncertainty, no training and redeployment to unknown areas, wellness programmes were initiated [26]. These included free wellbeing classes yoga, Pilates or meditation, free food donations and greater awareness on media – seeking mental health services were thus more accessible as it was not seen as a weakness [26]. This depicts the benefits of social media.

## 7. Conclusions

The covid 19 pandemic thought us many lessons but we also used lessons from the past. Previous experience with MCIs assisted during the many different waves and variants. Ever changing PPE protocols and transmissibility of the virus showed us that we had more to learn and adapt. Globally we were not well prepared for this MCI as evidenced by Oxygen and ventilator shortages as well as the strain on our human resources by health care personnel burn out. The greatest lesson learnt is the versatility of the medical professional, assisting in areas they are not specialized in (surgeons in infectious disease wards and critical care settings of intensivist), redistributing resources with ever changing protocols. Although there was a global response to the front line to treat patients of a MCI, the amount of research and literature churned out by clinicians is impressive. This will serve as the foundation for future pandemics/ MCIs, and one would hope that it will not be as prolonged as the current pandemic.

## Conflict of interest

The author declare no conflict of interest.

## Author details

Naadiyah Laher[1,2*]

1 Faculty of Health Sciences, Department of Surgery, School of Clinical Medicine, University of the Witwatersrand, Johannesburg, South Africa

2 Charlotte Maxeke Johannesburg Academic Hospital Trauma Unit and Chris Hani Baragwanath Academic Hospital Trauma Unit, Johannesburg, South Africa

*Address all correspondence to: naadiyahlaher@gmail.com

## References

[1] American College of Surgeons. Initial assessment and management. In: *Advanced Trauma Life Support*. Chicago: American College of Surgeons; 2018

[2] CDC. Centre for disease control and prevention. 4 November 2021 [Online]. Available from: https://www.cdc.gov/coronavirus/2019-ncov/hcp/non-us-settings/emergency-considerations-ppe.html [Accessed: January 21, 2022]

[3] Lewis D. Covid 19 rarely infects through surfaces. So why are we still deep cleaning? Nature. 2021;**590**:26-28

[4] Dong E, Du H, Gardner L. An interactive web-based dashboard to track COVID-19 in real time. The Lancet Infectious Diseases. 2020;**20**(5):533-534

[5] Okoye O. Implementing trauma resuscitation protocol in COVID 19 era: Our modifications at the National Trauma Centre, Abuja, Nigeria. *Nigerian Journal of Clinical Practice*. 2021;**24**(**1**):138-141

[6] Gómez-Ochoa SA, Franco OH, Rojas LZ, Raguindin PF, Roa-Diaz ZM, et al. COVID-19 in health-care workers: A living systematic review and Meta-analysis of prevalence, risk factors, clinical characteristics, and outcomes. American Journal of Epidemiology. 2021;**190**(1):161-175, erratum 187

[7] Livingstone DH, Bonne S, Morello C, Fox A. Optimizing the trauma resuscitation bay during the Covid-19 pandemic. Trauma Surgery & Acute Care Open. 2020;**5**:1-3

[8] Howard BE. High-risk aerosol-generating procedures in COVID-19: Respiratory protective equipment considerations. Otolaryngology–Head and Neck Surgery. 2020;**163**(**1**):98-103

[9] Ponnappan KT, Sam AF, Tempe DK, Arora MK. Intubation box in the current pandemic - helps or hinders? Anaesthesia, Critical Care & Pain Medicine. 2020;**39**(**5**):587-588

[10] Davies M, Hodzovic I. Videolaryngoscopy post COVID-19. Trends in Anaesthesia & Critical Care. 2021;**36**:49-51

[11] Ludwin K, Bialka Z, Czyzewski L, Smereka J, Dabrowski M, et al. Video laryngoscopy for endotracheal intubation of adult patients with suspected/confirmed COVID-19. A systematic review and meta-analysis of randomized controlled trials. Disaster and Emergency Medicine Journal. 2020;**5**(**2**):85-97

[12] Olding J, Zisman S, Olding C, Fan K. Penetrating trauma during a global pandemic: Changing patterns in interpersonal violence, self-harm and domestic violence in the Covid-19 outbreak. The Surgeon. 2021;**19**:E9-E13

[13] Tankel J, Einav S. Preparing for mass casualty events despite COVID-19. British Journal of Anaesthesia. 2022;**128**(2):e104-e108

[14] WHO. Mass Casualty Management Systems: Strategies and Guidelines for Buidling Health Sector Capacity. Geneva: WHO; 2007

[15] Coccolini F, Sartelli M, Kluger Y, Pikoulis E, Karamagioli E, et al. COVID-19 the showdown for mass casualty preparedness and management: The Cassandra syndrome. World Journal of Emergency Surgery. 2020;**15**(**26**):1-6

[16] MSF. Relief web. OCHA. 11 May 2021 [Online]. Available from: https://reliefweb.int/report/world/

gasping-air-deadly-shortages-medical-oxygen-covid-19-patients-msf-briefing-paper-may [Accessed: January 22, 2022]

[17] Leo CG, Sabina S, Tumolo MR, Bodini A, Ponzini G, et al. Burnout among healthcare workers in the COVID 19 era: A review of the existing literature. Frontiers in Public Health. 2021;**9**:1-6. DOI: 10.3389/fpubh.2021.750529

[18] Ziblim A, Sumeghy MG, Cartwright A. The dynamics of informal settlements upgrading in South Africa. Habitat International. 2013;**37**:316-334

[19] Hau HM, Weitz J, Bork U. Impact of the COVID-19 pandemic on student and resident teaching and training in surgical oncology. Journal of Clinical Medicine. 2020;**9**(**11**):3431

[20] Liang ZC, Ooi SBS, Wang W. Pandemics and their impact on medical training: Lessons from Singapore. Academic Medicine. 2020;**95**(**9**):1359-1361

[21] e. H. R. T. Force. "ems.gov." 05 June 2020 [Online]. Available from: https://www.ems.gov/pdf/Federal_Guidance_and_Resources/Patient_Care/Interim_Guidance_Field_Trauma_Triage_Principles.pdf [Accessed: January 22, 2022]

[22] Editorial. Palliative care and the COVID-19 pandemic. Lancet. 2020;**395**:1168

[23] Elster E, Potter BK, Chung K. Response to COVID-19 by the surgical community. Surgery. 2020;**167**:907-908

[24] A. ASA. American society of anaesthesiologist. 8 December 2020 [Online]. Available from: https://www.asahq.org/about-asa/newsroom/news-releases/2020/12/asa-and-apsf-joint-statement-on-elective-surgery-and-anesthesia-for-patients-after-covid-19-infection [Accessed: January 22, 2022]

[25] Giangola M, Siskind S, Faliks B, Dela Cruz R, Lee A, et al. Applying triage principles of mass casualty events to the SARS-CoV-2 pandemic: From the perspective of the acute care surgeons at Long Island Jewish medical Center in the COVID epicenter of the United States. Surgery. 2020;**168**:408-410

[26] Tahmassebi R, Bates P, Trompeter A, Bhattacharya R, El-Daly I, et al. Reflections from London's Level-1 major trauma centres. European Journal of Orthopaedic Surgery and Traumatology. 2020;**30**:951-954

Chapter 5

# ICU Management of Tetanus

*Ballah Abubakar, Jacob Dunga, Yusuf B. Jibrin, Hassan Maina, Bordiya G. Buma and Ibrahim Maigari*

## Abstract

Tetanus is a major public health concern in low socio economic countries and it carries a high mortality rate. However, the incidence of tetanus in developed nations has greatly reduced due to an excellent vaccine program. Tetanus is caused by a neurotoxin released by *Clostridium tetani*. *C. tetani* is a spore-forming bacterium that is widely distributed in soil and it is also found in the intestines and feces of animals such as horses, sheep, cattle, dogs, cats, rats and guinea pigs. The mortality is because of various complications due to muscle spasms, autonomic dysfunction, as well as due to prolonged critical care. Management of tetanus with its complications is in an intensive care unit and the goals of management include stopping further toxin production, neutralization of unbound toxin, management of the airway, control of muscle spasm, treatment of autonomic dysfunction and general supportive management. The effective method of preventing tetanus is by immunization with tetanus toxoid containing vaccines. The vaccine is cheap, effective and safe for all age groups.

**Keywords:** tetanus, rigidity, seizures, spasms, benzodiazepines, magnesium sulphate, intensive care unit, mechanical ventilation

## 1. Introduction

Tetanus is an acute, potentially fatal disease that is characterized by generalized increased rigidity and convulsive spasms of skeletal muscles. It is caused by a neurotoxin released by *Clostridium tetani*. *C. tetani* is a spore-forming bacterium that is widely distributed in soil and it is also found in the intestines and feces of animals such as horses, sheep, cattle, dogs, cats, rats and guinea pigs. Agriculturally, soil treated with manure may contain large numbers of spores also. In agricultural areas due to soil treatment with manure, a significant number of human adults may harbor the organism too. It enters the body through breaks in the skin and germinates under anaerobic conditions [1]. Tetanus is a vaccine-preventable disease that remains a common cause of acute critical illness in low-income and middle-income countries (LMICs). It is estimated that the annual mortality of tetanus is around 200,000–300,000 with over a half of these deaths found in neonates. Neonatal tetanus is a severe, often fatal disease caused by a toxin of *C. tetani*. The World Health Organization defines a confirmed case of neonatal tetanus as an illness in a child who has normal feeding and crying during the first 2 days of life but loses the ability between age 3 and 28 days of life and becomes rigid and has spasms. It occurs through infection of the umbilicus when the cord is cut with an unclean instrument or when substances heavily contaminated with tetanus spores are applied to the umbilical stump. Infants who have not acquired passive immunity from the mother because she has not been immunized are at an increased risk. Tetanus is however relatively rare in the developed world. Where they occur, it is usually in the adult. Neonatal tetanus has been eliminated in Europe [2].

## 2. Pathophysiology

The *C. tetani* bacterium is a spore-forming, gram-positive, slender, anaerobic rod. It is heat sensitive and cannot survive in the presence of oxygen. The spores however are extremely resistant to heat and they can survive autoclaving at a temperature up to 121°C for 10–15 min. The spores of *C. tetani* are widely distributed in the environment and they reside in soil, faeces and dust. Once the spores enter the body through a wound, they germinate in the presence of an anaerobic condition. In some patients, no entry site is seen. Spores of *C. tetani* can also gain entry into the body through burns, surgery sites or childbirth. It has an incubation period of 2 and 21 days with an average 8 days. The further the injury site is from the central nervous system the longer the incubation period. Shorter incubation periods are associated with severe form of the disease and a higher chance of death. *C. tetani* produces two exotoxins, tetanolysin and tetanospasmin. Tetanospasmin is a neurotoxin and it is responsible for the clinical presentations of tetanus. This is an extremely potent neurotoxin and it is estimated that the minimum human lethal dose is 2.5 ng/kg of body weight (a nanogram is one billionth of a gram). The toxin spreads into the nervous system by binding to the neuromuscular junction and then being transported backwards into the cell body. Further spread occurs trans-synaptically to adjacent motor and autonomic nerves. The effect of tetanospasmin is by cleaving synaptobrevin which is a vesicle-associated membrane protein which is essential for the release of neurotransmitter. The inhibitory pathways is the most affected there by preventing the release of glycine and g-amino butyric acid (GABA). When interneurones inhibiting alpha motor neurones are affected, there is failure to inhibit motor reflexes [3]. This causes increased muscle tone and rigidity, interposed by sudden and potentially devastating muscle spasms. Muscles of the face are affected early because of their short axonal pathways. Sympathetic neurones become affected later in the disease. Disinhibited autonomic discharge leads to loss of autonomic control, resulting in sympathetic overactivity and increased catecholamine levels. Neuronal binding of the toxin is irreversible. Recovery requires the growth of new nerve terminals, which explains the prolonged duration of the disease.

## 3. Diagnosis

The diagnosis of tetanus is clinical. History of vaccination, physical examination, signs and symptoms of muscle spasm, rigidity and pain are pointers to presence of tetanus. There are currently no confirmatory laboratory tests. The triad of muscle rigidity, muscle spasms and autonomic instability indicates the presence of the disease.

## 4. Clinical features

On the basis of clinical findings, four different forms of tetanus have been described.

1. Generalised tetanus

2. Localised tetanus

3. Cephalic tetanus

4. Neonatal tetanus

### 4.1 Generalised tetanus

Generalized tetanus is the most common form of tetanus accounting for up to 80% of reported cases. It attacks muscles throughout the entire body. Generalized tetanus attacks and inhibits mostly the motor neurons of the CNS and later the neurons of the ANS as well thereby presenting with a descending pattern with uncontrollable muscle contraction affecting muscles of the face and jaw (trismus or locked jaw) being the first sign followed by stiffness of the neck, difficulty in swallowing, and rigidity of abdominal muscles. Other symptoms include elevated temperature, sweating, elevated blood pressure, and episodic rapid heart rate. Spasms may occur frequently and can last for several minutes. Spasms continue for 3–4 weeks. Complete recovery may take months.

### 4.2 Localised tetanus

Localized tetanus is an uncommon form of the disease in which patients have persistent contraction of muscles in the same anatomic area as the injury. It is most commonly confined to the extremities. These contractions may persist for many weeks before gradually subsiding. Localized tetanus may precede the onset of generalized tetanus but is generally milder.

### 4.3 Cephalic tetanus

Cephalic tetanus is rare, and results from head injuries or otitis media in which *C. tetani* is present in the flora of the middle ear or following injuries to the head. There is involvement of the cranial nerves, especially in the facial area and patients may present with facial nerve palsies. The infection may become generalized.

### 4.4 Neonatal tetanus

Neonatal tetanus is a form of generalized tetanus that occurs in newborn infants born without protective passive immunity because the mother is not immune. It results in high mortality in developing countries and is responsible for up to 50% of death due to tetanus. The infection usually arises from contamination of the umbilical cord during unsanitary delivery practices, absent maternal vaccination and unhygienic cultural practices such as the application of cow dung to the umbilical stump during the neonatal period. In neonatal tetanus, symptoms usually appear from 4 to 14 days after birth, averaging about 7 days [4].

Generally, symptoms of tetanus can be summarized to include neck stiffness, sore throat, dysphagia and trismus. Muscle spasms are extremely painful and can cause tendon to rupture, joint dislocation and bone fractures. Spasm that extends to the facial muscles causes the typical facial expression known as *risus sardonicus*. Truncal spasm causes *opisthotonus*. Severe hypoventilation and life-threatening apnoea may occur during prolonged spasms. Hypertension and tachycardia occur mainly from increased sympathetic tone. Autonomic storms are associated with raised catecholamine levels. These alternate with episodes of sudden hypotension, bradycardia and asystole. Other features of autonomic disturbance include salivation, sweating, increased bronchial secretions, hyperpyrexia, gastric stasis and ileus [5].

## 5. Complications of tetanus

The complications of tetanus result from muscle spasm, autonomic dysfunction, and prolonged critical illness. All systems of the body are involved.

### 5.1 Respiratory system

Life threatening complications from involvement of the respiratory system include but not limited to apnoea, hypoxia, respiratory failure, laryngeal spasm, atelectasis, aspiration pneumonitis, etc. Prolonged ventilation may lead to ventilator associated pneumonia (VAP) and complications from tracheostomy e.g. tracheal stenosis. Breathing problems occur from tightening of vocal cords and muscle rigidity.

### 5.2 Cardiovascular system

The cardiovascular complications are from autonomic dysfunction and are the most serious complications. These include tachycardia, hypertension, ischaemia, hypotension, bradycardia, tachyarrhythmias, bradyarrhythmias, Asystole, heart failure. The pathogenesis is said to be due excessively high levels of circulating catecholamines.

Other complication related to the renal and gastrointestinal systems include; high output renal failure, Oliguric renal failure from rhabdomyolysis, urinary stasis, urinary tract infection, gastric stasis, ileus, diarrhoea, haemorrhage. Thromboembolism and skin breakdown has been reported. Dislocation of the temporomandibular and shoulder joints have also been reported. Sepsis with multiple organ failures can also occur with the progression of the disease.

## 6. Severity grading/prognosis

The Ablett classification of severity is the most commonly used grading system. It grades tetanus infection from mild (Grade I) to very severe (Grade IV) [6]. Prognosis

| Grade | Characteristics |
|---|---|
| Grade 1 (mild) | Mild trismus, general spasticity, no respiratory compromise, no spasms, no dysphagia |
| Grade 2 (moderate) | Moderate trismus, rigidity, short spasms, mild dysphagia, moderate respiratory involvement, ventilatory frequency >30 |
| Grade 3 (severe) | Severe trismus, generalized rigidity, prolonged spasms, severe dysphagia, apnoeic spells, pulse >120, ventilatory frequency >40 |
| Grade 4 (very severe) | Grade 3 with severe autonomic instability involving the cardiovascular system Severe hypertension and tachycardia, alternating with relative hypotension and bradycardia, either of which may be persistent |

**Table 1.**
*Ablett classification of severity.*

| Prognostic factor | Score 1 | Score 0 |
|---|---|---|
| Incubation period | <7 days | >7 days or unknown |
| Period of onset | <2 days | >2 days |
| Entry site | Umbilicus, burn, uterine, open fracture, surgical wound, intramuscular injection | All others plus unknown |
| Spasms | Present | absent |
| Fever | >38.4°C | <38.4°C |
| Tachycardia | Neonate > 150 beats/min<br>Adult > 120 beats/min | Neonate < 150 beats/min<br>Adult < 120 beats/min |
| Total score | | |

**Table 2.**
*Prognostic scoring systems in tetanus: Dakar score.*

| Score | Severity | Mortality |
|---|---|---|
| 0–1 | Mild | <10% |
| 2–3 | Moderate | 10–20% |
| 4 | Severe | 20–40% |
| 5–6 | Very severe | >50 |

**Table 3.**
*Total score, severity and disease prognosis.*

| **Incubation time:** | |
|---|---|
| <48 h | |
| 2–5 days | 4 |
| 5–10 days | 3 |
| 10–14 days | 2 |
| >14 days | 1 |
| Site of infection: | |
| Internal and umbilical | 5 |
| Head, neck, and body wall | 4 |
| Peripheral proximal | 3 |
| Peripheral distal | 2 |
| Unknown | 1 |
| State of protection: | |
| None 10 | 10 |
| Possibly some or maternal immunisation in neonatal patients | 8 |
| Protected > 10 years ago | 4 |
| Protected < 10 years ago | 2 |
| Complete protection | 0 |
| Complicating factors: | |
| Injury or life threatening illness 10 | 10 |

| Incubation time: | |
|---|---|
| Severe injury or illness not immediately life threathening | 8 |
| Injury or non-life threatening illness 4 | 4 |
| Minor injury or illness 2 | 2 |
| ASA grade 1 | 0 |
| Total | |
| *Mild <9, moderate 9–16, severe >16.* | |

**Table 4.**
*Prognostic scoring systems in tetanus: Phillips score*

is assessed using the Phillips score and the Dakar score. Both these scoring systems are relatively straightforward schemes which take into account the incubation period and the period of onset as well as presence of neurological and cardiac manifestations. The Phillips score also factors in the state of immune protection (**Tables 1–4**).

## 7. Management

There is currently no treatment for tetanus. Management of the disease requires an emergency and long term supportive care. Three strategic principles apply however apply.

- Neutralization of the toxin that is already in the body
- Destroying the organisms in the body to prevent further toxin release
- Minimizing the effects of the toxin already in the body

### 7.1 Neutralizing toxin already in the body

Intravenous human tetanus immunoglobulin (HTIG) 150 units/kg intramuscularly is used to neutralize free circulating toxin before it binds to neuronal cell membrane. The HTIG is an effective therapy and it is given as soon as the diagnosis of tetanus is considered. There is available an intravenous preparation of 5000–10,000 IU. HTIG is a specific solvent-detergent-treated plasma derived product obtained from donors immunized with tetanus toxoids. An initial skin sensitivity testing using a dose of 3000–6000 units intramuscularly is given. This drug does not neutralize intracellular toxin which is already fixed to the nerve terminals. HTIG is contraindicated in patients with history of anaphylactic reaction to the active substance or to any of the component of the product. Also patients with deficiency of mmunoglobulin A and the intramuscular test dose is contraindicated in those with severe thrombocytopenia or any coagulation disorder.

#### *7.1.1 Airway management*

Respiratory failure has been identified as the commonest direct cause of death from tetanus in the less developed world. This may not be unconnected with lack of ventilator support where it is needed. The Intensivist should anticipate patients at risk of hypoxia and airways obstruction, aspiration hypoventilation, pneumonia, and respiratory arrest. Such patients should be closely monitored and connected to ventilator support as soon as possible. Early airways protection initially with endotracheal tube or tracheostomy is often needed. Ventilator modes used depends on complexity of the ventilators available in the intensive care unit. In the early stages of the disease when rigidity and spasm are prominent, sedation, analgesia and muscular paralysis are required to allow for controlled mandatory ventilation. This mode usually provides rest to the already fatigue muscles of respiration. It is important to note that the controlled mandatory ventilation mode is used only when necessary. Poor lung compliance and oxygenation due to muscular rigidity or pulmonary complications may be overcome by a combination of pressure controlled ventilation and positive end expiratory pressure (PEEP). In the later stages of the disease, modes of ventilation that allow spontaneous ventilation (synchronised intermittent mandatory, continuous positive airway pressure and biphasic positive airway pressure ventilation) are generally preferred and may optimize the respiratory pattern, reduce sedation requirements, minimise muscle wastage, and reduce the likelihood of acquired critical illness neuropathy or myopathy. Mechanical ventilation is better and more comforting for the patient if a tracheostomy is given early. Tracheostomy increases patients comfort, reduced dead space and airway resistance with reduced risk of airway trauma especially in patients convulsing. Endotracheal intubation has been associated with more complications such as subglottic stenosis, vocal cord immobility, laryngeal granuloma, need for deeper sedation when compared to tracheostomy and higher mortality rate. Sedation is an essential component of the management of tetanus patients being ventilated in ICU. It is required to relieve the discomfort and anxiety caused by airway manipulation, ventilation, suction and physiotherapy. Sedation can also minimize agitation yet maximize rest and appropriate sleep. Analgesia is an almost universal requirement for ventilated patients. Combination of opioids and benzodiazepines used for controlling seizures in tetanus gives a good outcome. Adequate sedation and analgesia ameliorates the stress response to tracheal intubation and mechanical ventilation.

### 7.2 Destroy the organisms in the body to prevent further toxin release

Metronidazole is used to destroy the organisms in the body. It diffuses into the organism and inhibits its protein synthesis by interacting with DNA and causes loss of helical DNA structure. A dose of 30–40 mg/kg/day in three divided doses for children and 0.5 g three times daily for up to 10 days is recommended. Other drugs that are effective include Penicillin G (100,000–200,000 IU/kg/day intravenously, given in four divided doses). Macrolides such as erythromycin given as 30–50 mg/kg/day in three divided doses for children and 0.5 g/kg/day in three divided doses for adults has shown effectiveness. Tetracyclines, clindamycin, cephalosporins and chloramphenicol are also effective. To reduce further bacterial load and toxin, if a wound responsible for tetanus is clear, thorough cleaning of infected site with extensive surgical debridement is recommended if patient is stable. Surgical debridement helps to eradicate spores and necrotic tissues which could lead to conditions ideal for germination. To reduce the risk of releasing tetanospasmin into the bloog stream, it is advised that wound manipulation should be delayed until hours after administration of antitoxin.

### 7.3 Minimise the effects of the toxin already in the body

Circulating tetanus toxins cause muscle rigidity, spasm and autonomic instability. Treatment of rigidity and spasm is very effective in preventing exhaustion, respiratory failure, aspiration pneumonitis and dysphagia. Spasm and rigidity can be treated effectively with sedation and limiting unnecessary stimulation. Benzodiazepine along or in combination with other drugs such as anticonvulsants have been used with great successes. The first line of treatment is the benzodiazepines.

Diazepam one of the derivative of benzodiazepines and is very effective in tetanus management. It acts by increasing GABA agonism through resistance to endogenous inhibitors of the GABAA receptor. The benefits of diazepam are as anti-convulsant and muscle relaxant that acts to control rigidity and muscle spasms. In addition, diazepam has sedative and anxiolytic effects. Large doses up to 100 mg/h can be administered and may cause mild respiratory depression.

Midazolam, also a benzodiazepine can be used in the absence of Diazepam. It is however relatively short-acting. Morphine can be equally efficacious and is usually used as an adjunct to benzodiazepine sedation.

Propofol has also been used successfully with rapid recovery occurring once the infusion is stopped however, in order to achieve adequate plasma concentrations to relieve muscle rigidity, mechanical ventilation is necessary.

In a patient with tetanus on mechanical ventilation, neuromuscular blocking agents can be used to control the muscle spasm if it continues despite the use of sedatives. Vecuronium is a short-acting neuromuscular blocker. It has minimal cardiovascular effects and does not release histamines. The use of pancuronium and atracurium is not recommended because pancuronium causes tachycardia while atracurium causes bradycardia and hypotension which may trigger mortality in the patient with tetanus. Newer agents such as pipercuronium and rocuronium are long acting and provide good haemodynamic stability they are however expensive compared with older drugs.

Anticonvulsants such as phenobarbitone, (which enhances GABA activity) and phenothiazine such as and chlorpromazine may be used to provide additional sedation. When sedation alone is inadequate, neuromuscular blocking agents and intermittent positive pressure ventilation may be required, usually for a prolonged period.

Baclofen is a structural analogue of $GABA_B$ receptor agonist that inhibits presynaptic acetylcholine release and synaptic medullar reflexes. These effects help in an anti-spastic action. They act by lowering calcium permeability in primary afferents. Intrathecal administration of 500-2000μg daily of baclofen had caused decrease muscle spasm in generalised tetanus [7].

### 7.4 Autonomic instability

Circulatory collapse is a major cause of mortality in tetanus and this is caused by autonomic instability. Sudden cardiac arrest is common and is thought to be precipitated by a combination of high catecholamine levels and the direct action of the tetanus toxin on the myocardium. Prolonged sympathetic activity may end with profound hypotension and bradycardia. Parasympathetic over activity may lead to sinus arrest. Direct damage to the vagal nucleus by the tetanus toxin has been implicated. Sedation with Benzodiazepines, anticonvulsant medication and morphine is the first line maneuver to control autonomic instability and also magnesium sulphate has been used as a preventive measure with success.

Magnesium sulfate is a pre-synaptic neuromuscular blocker. It inhibits catecholamine release from nerves and adrenal medulla and also reduces receptor responsiveness to released catecholamines, anticonvulsants, and vasodilators. Magnesium sulphate is a calcium antagonist in the myocardium and neuromuscular junction and inhibits the release of parathyroid hormone thereby decreasing calcium levels. Doses are initiated with loading dose 75–80 mg/kg in 30 min and followed by 2 g/h in patients under 60 years and 1 g/h for patients over 60 years. Morphine is very useful in maintaining cardiovascular stability. The mechanism of action of morphine includes replacement of endogenous opioids, reduction of sympathetic reflex activity and histamine release [8]. Phenothiazine especially chlorpromazine which acts as anticholinergic and $\alpha$ adrenergic antagonism also play a role in maintaining cardiovascular stability and used as a sedative.

B-blockade, although theoretically useful to control episodes of hypertension and tachycardia, is associated with sudden cardiovascular collapse, pulmonary oedema and death.

### 7.5 Supportive care

Patients with tetanus suffer weight loss due to several factors. These include inability to swallow, autonomic induced alterations in gastrointestinal function, increased metabolic rate due to pyrexia and muscular activity from convulsion and seizure. Nutrition should therefore be established as early as possible. Due to trismus, oral feeding is not possible. Nasogastric tube should be passed as early as possible to commence feeding. High caloric nutritional supplement is required to meet the high metabolic demand of tetanus. Parenteral nutrition is preferred but it is expensive and majority of tetanus patients are from a poor socio-economic status.

Nosocomial infection such as VAP is common among critically ill patients that are ventilated. The prevalence of VAP is a common indicator for safety and quality of care in critically ill patients admitted to the ICU. This is associated with increased mortality among ventilated patients. Measures taken to prevent VAP include strict hand hygiene with alcohol solutions before airway management, continuous aspiration of subglottic secretions, oral hygiene with chlorhexidine, semi recumbent positioning of patients where possible and selective decontamination of the digestive tract or selective oropharyngeal decontamination.

Venous thromboembolism (VTE) is a common and major complication in the critically ill patients. The use of intermittent pneumatic compression or graduated compression stockings with regular turning of patient help to prevent thromboembolism.

Other supportive measures foot drop splint to prevent ankle contracture, limb and chest physiotherapy, regular turning of patient or use of air/water mattress to prevent decubitus ulcer, care of the patient should be in dark room with minimal stimulus and psychosocial support.

## 8. Prevention

The effective method of preventing tetanus is by immunization with tetanus toxoid containing vaccines. The vaccine is cheap, effective and safe for all age groups. In children, three doses are given from as early as six weeks of life and repeated at intervals of 4 weeks. It is also advised that three booster doses are given to confer lifelong immunity. It is also administered to pregnant women during pregnancy as a part of ante natal care package and also women in the reproductive age groups. To maintain high level of protection, individuals with cuts and open wound are given the tetanus toxoid containing vaccine [9].

## 9. Conclusion

Tetanus is a vaccine preventable disease but it has remained a public health problem in developing countries mostly due to poor vaccine coverage, poverty and low levels of education. All wounds other than clean minor ones should be considered tetanus prone therefore, HTIG should be considered. The diagnosis of tetanus is clinical and it can be fatal if missed. The mortality rate of tetanus is high and prolonged ICU care may be required. The outcome depends on early diagnosis, identification and management of complications and a good supportive care which the patient receives.

## Author details

Ballah Abubakar[1*], Jacob Dunga[2], Yusuf B. Jibrin[3], Hassan Maina[4], Bordiya G. Buma[5] and Ibrahim Maigari[3]

1 Department of Anaesthesia and ICU, Atbu Teaching Hospital, Bauchi State, Nigeria

2 Respiratory Unit, Internal Medicine Department, Atbu Teaching Hospital, Bauchi State, Nigeria

3 Infectious Disease Unit, Internal Medicine Department, Atbu Teaching Hospital, Bauchi State, Nigeria

4 Department of Anaesthesia and ICU, Federal Medical Center, Yola, Adamawa State, Nigeria

5 Department of Anaesthesia and ICU, Federal Medical Center, Jalingo, Taraba, Nigeria

*Address all correspondence to: abubakarballah196@gmail.com; mballah@atbu.edu.ng

## References

[1] Olum S, Eyul J, Lukwiya DO, Scolding N. Tetanus in a rural low-income intensive care unit setting. Brain Communications. 2021;**3**(1)

[2] Kyu HH, Mumford JE, Stanaway JD, Barber RM, Hancock JR, et al. Mortality from tetanus between 1990 and 2015: Findings from the global burden of disease study 2015. BMC Public Health. 2017;**17**:179

[3] Cook TM, Protheroe RT, Handel JM. Tetanus: A review of the literature. British Journal of Anaesthesia. 2001;**87**:477-487

[4] Sathirapanya P, Sathirapanya C, Limapichat K, Setthawacharawanich S, Phabphal K. Tetanus: A retrospective study of clinical presentations and outcomes in a medical teaching hospital. Journal of the Medical Association of Thailand. 2009;**92**:315-319

[5] Govindaraj GM, Riyaz A. Current practice in the management of tetanus. *Critical Care*. 2014;**18**:145

[6] Ablett JJL. Analysis and main experiences in 82 patients treated in the Leeds Tetanus Unit. In: Ellis M, editor. Symposium on Tetanus in Great Britain. Boston Spa, UK: Leeds General Infirmary; 1967. pp. 1-10

[7] Rodrigo C, Fernando D, Rajapakse S. Pharmacological management of tetanus: an evidence-based review. *Critical Care*. 2014;**18**:217

[8] Mathew PJ, Samra T, Wig J. Magnesium sulphate for treatment of tetanus in adults. Anaesthesia and Intensive Care. 2010;**38**:185-189

[9] WHO. 2010. Current recommendations for treatment of tetanus during humanitarian emergencies. Available from: http://www.who.int/diseasecontrol_emergencies/who_hse_gar_dce_2010_en.pdf

Chapter 6

# Protocols for Bleeding and Thrombosis in Pediatric Intensive Care Units

*Rungrote Natesirinilkul*

## Abstract

Bleeding and thrombosis are the common hematological complications found in children who are admitted in the pediatric intensive care units (PICUs). Some of those complications could be mild, however some could be serious or life-threatening for critically-ill children. The etiologies of those conditions could be due to the underlying diseases, i.e., congenital bleeding disorders, complications of the diseases, i.e. coagulopathy due to disseminated intravascular coagulation (DIC), and also the side effects from the treatments themselves, i.e., massive transfusion or extracorporeal membrane oxygenation (ECMO). Early detection and management and prevention of those complications could decrease the morbidity and mortality of the children in PICUs. Although most guidelines of management of those bleeding and thrombosis in adults is well established, the evidences for the management of those conditions in children are limited. In addition, developmental hemostasis during the childhood, which is different from adulthood, could challenge the management of those conditions in children admitted in PICUs.

**Keywords:** pediatrics, intensive care unit, massive transfusion, extracorporeal membrane oxygenation, thromboprophylaxis

## 1. Introduction

Pediatric patients who are admitted in pediatric intensive care units (PICUs) are at risk of having bleeding and thrombotic complications due to several factors including their underlying diseases, the medications and procedures they received during the admission and the current conditions of the patients that lead them to be admitted in PICUs [1]. Since the hemostasis in children are different from the adults, management of bleeding and thrombosis in pediatric patients is challenging and may not be directly adopted from the evidences in adult patients. Moreover, developmental hemostasis should be taken into accounts of management. This chapter includes massive transfusion, extracorporeal oxygen membrane oxygenation (ECMO) and venous thromboembolism (VTE) protocols in children based on current evidences.

## 2. Developmental hemostasis

The hemostasis is a group of system which is responsible for the bleeding control after a vascular injury and also recanalization of that vessel when the bleeding is stopped. The balance between the bleeding control, which is the interaction between primary and secondary hemostatic systems, and the recanalization process, including anticoagulation and fibrinolytic systems, is crucial to maintain normal hemostasis in the body [2, 3]. The summary of normal hemostatic system is shown in **Figure 1**. The defects in the bleeding control cause bleeding disorders while the impairment of recanalization process lead to thrombotic disorders.

As same as other systems in the human body, the hemostatic system has been changed from the neonatal period to the adulthood in all parts of hemostatic system. The summary of developmental changes in hemostatic system in summarized in **Table 1**.

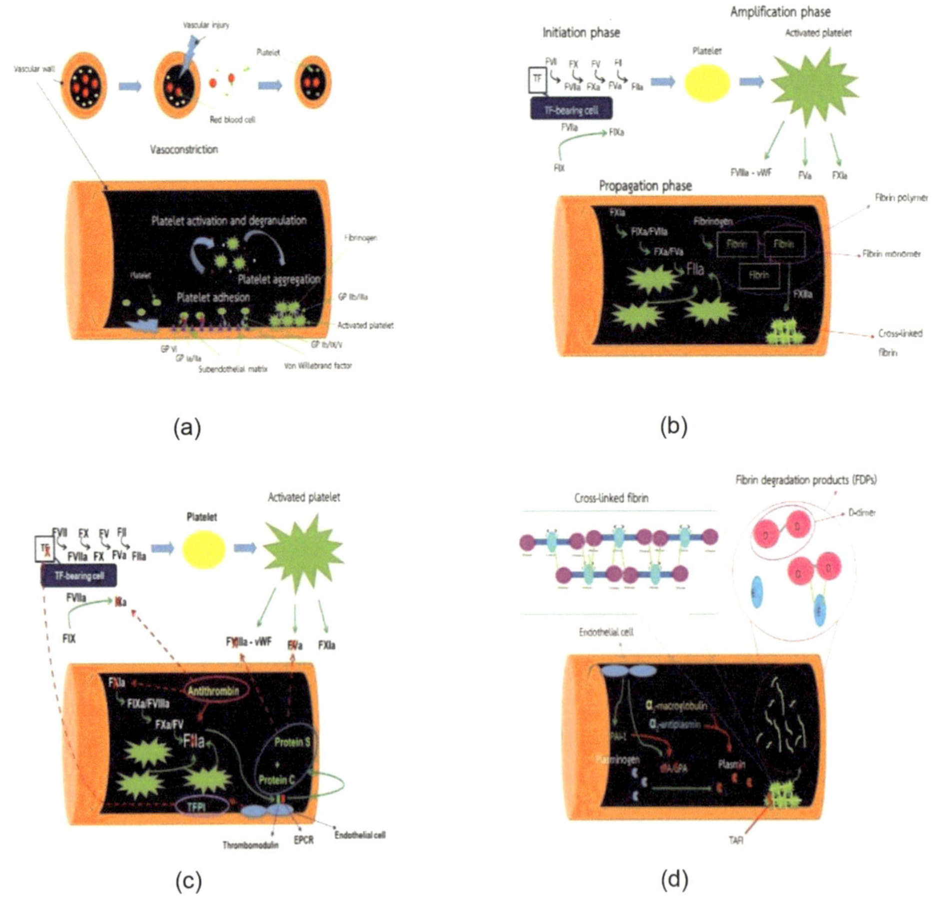


**Figure 1.**
*The summary of normal hemostatic system. (a). Primary hemostasis. (b). Secondary hemostasis. (c). Anticoagulation system. (d). Fibrinolytic system.*

| Hemostatic system | Comparison between children and adults |
|---|---|
| Primary hemostatic system | • *Vessel wall and endothelial cells:*<br>o Elevated glycoaminoglycans in vessels of neonates leading to increased antithrombotic property by working with antithrombin (AT)<br>o Increased von Willebrand factor (VWF) and large VWF multimers from endothelial cells<br>• *Platelets:*<br>o Platelet numbers in term neonates = those in children and adults but may decrease in preterm neonates<br>o Platelets in term neonates express low receptors on platelet surface resulting in less platelet response<br>o High red cell mass, mean corpuscular volume (MCV), VWF and elevated proportion of large VWF multimers |
| Secondary hemostatic system | • Vitamin K-dependent factors (prothrombin, FVII, FIX and FX), contact factors and FV < adult levels<br>• FVIII, VWF and tissue factor (TF) levels > adults in first 6 months of life<br>• Fibrinogen, FV and FXIII = adult levels |
| Anticoagulation system | • Protein C (PC), protein S (PS), AT and tissue factor pathway inhibitor (TFPI) < adult levels |
| Fibrinolysis system | • Plasmin, plasminogen activator inhibitor (PAI)-1 and $\alpha_2$-antiplasmin (AP) < adult levels<br>• tissue plasminogen activator (t-PA) and $\alpha_2$-macroglobulin (M) > in adult levels |
| Net hemostasis | • Endogenous thrombin potential (ETP) almost 2-time in neonates than adults |

**Table 1.**
*The summary of developmental changes of hemostasis [4, 5].*

## 2.1 Massive transfusion protocol in children

In adult patients who undergo major surgeries or experience traumas, massive transfusion is defined by transfusion of blood components particularly red blood cell concentrate (RBC) equal or more than 10 units within 24 hours, receiving RBC more than 4 units in 1 hour or requirement of blood components more than 50% of total blood volume within 3 hours [6]. Although the definition of massive transfusion in children is unclear, some studies defined receiving transfusion volume of blood components more than 40 ml/kg within 24 hours as massive transfusion [7]. Moreover, adoption of adult's definitions of massive transfusion is not practical in pediatrics as some may not survive long enough to fit with those definitions. Moreover, Acker et al. showed that the adoption of assessment blood consumption (ABC) scale of adults in children had less sensitivity and specificity than those when it was studied in adult population [8]. Although the current proposed definition of pediatric massive transfusion is transfusion of blood components more than 37 ml/kg within 4 hours to make the diagnosis and initiate the intervention sooner [7], more studies are required to confirm the benefits of this definition.

The main mechanisms of massive transfusion consist of severe tissue injury from the surgery or trauma which releases abundant mount of tissue factor (TF) which massively activated coagulation cascades and hemodilution of the inappropriate resuscitation with intravenous fluid and blood components. Those subsequently lead to a vicious cycle of progressive coagulopathy, acidosis and hypothermia which results in ongoing bleeding and multiorgan failure [6].

When the pediatric patients reach the definition of massive transfusion, the activation of the massive transfusion protocol (MTP) should be commenced. Currently, most MTPs are driven by blood components ratio protocol. The common MTPs suggest 1:1:1 ratio of fresh frozen plasma (FFP): RBC: platelet concentrate (PC) [10]. However, the most effective ratio between FFP and RBC is still controversy. Cunningham et al. reported that high (≥ 1: 1) FFP: RBC ratio, associated with better survival outcome at 4 and 24 hours than medium (≥ 1:2 to <1:1) and low (< 1:2) FFP: RBC ratios (P = 0.02). The survival outcome of medium PC: RBC ratio was higher than high and low ratios of PC:RBC without statistical significance [9]. In addition, Diab et al. recommended ratio of FFP:RBC:PC or cryoprecipitate (cryo) at 1:1:2 for massive transfusion in children [6]. However, the systematic review by Maw and Furyk showed minimal benefit of fixed ratio of FFP: RBC: PC at 1:1:1 in pediatric massive transfusion [10]. Though all blood components are derived from the whole blood (WB), hematocrit, platelet count and coagulation factors are higher in WB and lower volume than each separated blood component [7]. Furthermore, a few studies showed faster access with similar safety and clinical outcomes of using WB for resuscitation in children [11, 12].

Besides fixed ratio of blood components protocol for massive transfusion, thromboelastography (TEG) and rotational thromboelastometry (ROTEM), the viscoelastic test to measure global hemostasis and currently used as a point-of-care testing [POCT], have been used as a guided tool for management of massive transfusion [7, 10, 13]. The systematic review of using TEG or ROTEM to measure hemostasis in adults and children revealed lower dose of transfused blood components and decreased mortality than the fixed ratio for massive transfusion in patients with bleeding [13].

Other adjunctive treatments of massive transfusion include tranexamic acid (TXA) and recombinant activated factor VII (rFVIIa). Tranexamic acid, a lysine analogue, is an antifibrinolytic agent which inhibits plasminogen activation and prevent fibrinolytic process [7]. The pediatric trauma and tranexamic acid study (PED-TRAX) revealed TXA significantly decreased mortality rate (odds ratio 0.3) without increasing thromboembolic (TE) and cardiovascular events in pediatric population [14]. rFVIIa, a bypassing agent, which is used for bleeding control in both hemophiliac A and B patients who have inhibitor to factor VIII and IX, respectively [15]. The systematic review by McQuilten et al. showed no benefit of the decreased mortality for the off-label use of rFVIIa in massive transfusion and there was an increased risk of TE, particularly arterial TE, in patients using rFVIIa, therefore, routinely using rFVIIa as a part of MTP is not recommended [16].

### 2.2 Extracorporeal oxygen membrane oxygenation (ECMO) protocol in children

ECMO is an equipment used for cardiopulmonary support in children who have severe cardiac and/or pulmonary compromise and do not respond to medications and mechanical ventilatory support. There are two types of ECMO, venovenous (VV) ECMO which mainly support respiratory system while venoarterial (VA) ECMO support both respiratory and cardiac system [17–19]. To maintain the blood flow of ECMO circuit, which is an artificial system with nonbiological surface, the usage of an anticoagulant, mainly unfractionated heparin (UFH), is required to reduce thrombin and fibrin formation in the ECMO circuit. The current guideline for ECMO management is recommended by Extracorporeal Life Support Organization (ELSO) registry which is the largest international adult and pediatric database for patients treated with extracorporeal life support (ECLS) [19]. There are four parts of ECMO circuit including a cannula, a pump with console, an oxygenator and a heart exchanger [20].

Monitoring and adjustment of the UFH dosage to balance between bleeding and clotting in patients using ECMO is challenging [21]. Dalton et al. reported the high bleeding complication in children receiving ECMO at 70% including 16% of intracranial bleeding. In contrast, 31% of children required ECMO circuit components changes due to clot and 13% of children developed patient-associated clot [22]. Although the standard dose of UFH for ECMO is the treatment dose of UFH at 20–25 unit/kg/hour, the variation of dose could be increased to 50–60 unit/kg/hour to reach the target ranges of UFH monitoring [23]. The summary of methods for UFH monitoring with the target ranges of each methods is shown in **Table 2**. However, the target ranges can be varied based on the institutional protocol, normal laboratory reference range of each test and the current bleeding conditions of the patients and thrombotic status of both patients and ECMO circuits. Moreover, there is currently no one perfect laboratory test to monitor UFH when the children are receiving ECMO.

Antithrombin (AT) is a natural anticoagulant and the main targeted protein working UFH to inhibit FXa and thrombin [23]. Therefore, the effect of heparin can be decreased by the deficiency of AT or heparin resistance particularly in infants aged less than 6 months when the synthesis of AT is not fully developed [21, 27]. Although the targeted AT level while the patients are receiving ECMO is approximately 70–120% [21, 28], there is no current consensus on that targeted AT level, the dosage, the timing and method of administration even in adult patients [28]. Moreover, the impact of AT supplementation in patients receiving ECMO is less understandable than that in patients with hereditary AT deficiency due to the patient and circuit interaction and their underlying diseases [21]. Furthermore, the widely available source of AT is FFP which is not appropriate source of AT and the AT concentrate, both plasma-derived and recombinant products with various properties of each product, can be accessible only in some countries [21].

In children who have contraindication of using UFH such as heparin-induced thrombocytopenia (HIT) or heparin resistance [21], bivalirudin, an intravenous direct thrombin inhibitor which inhibit both circulating thrombin and clot bound thrombin [29] could be an alternative anticoagulant for children receiving ECMO [23]. The median loading dose of bivalirudin is 0.1–0.125 mg/kg and the maintenance dose between 0.045 and 0.48 (0.125) mg/kg/hour [27, 30] to keep targeted APTT between 45 and 85 sec [23, 27]. However, unlike heparin, no antidote is available for bivalirudin and dose reduction is needed in children with renal disease as the main clearance organs are kidney and liver [23, 27].

### 2.3 Venous thromboembolism (VTE) prophylaxis in children

The incidence of VTE in children has been increasing during the last two decades in both Western and Asian countries especially in hospitalized children [31–33]. Even though the guideline for VTE thromboprophylaxis is well established in adult population [34, 35], the statement of VTE prophylaxis is not clearly mentioned with the limited available evidences and various details of the study [36–38].

Apart from pediatric patients who have hereditary thrombophilia, the hospitalized children are at risk of development of TE since two of three most common risk factors

| Methods | Blood sample for testing | Target ranges | Advantages | Drawbacks |
|---|---|---|---|---|
| Activated clotting time (ACT) | Whole blood | 150–170 sec | • POCT<br>• Less amount of required blood volume<br>• Measurement of whole blood clotting | • Difference between operator<br>• Specific to each analyzer and reagent<br>• Results interfered by platelet defects, other coagulopathy, hypothermia and hemodilution |
| Activated partial thromboplastin time (APTT) | Plasma | 60–90 sec<br>40–60 sec in patients with bleeding risk | • Widely available<br>• Ability to defect other etiologies of coagulopathy by using heparinase | • Specific to each analyzer, method of measurement and reagent<br>• Different normal reference range for age<br>• More amount of required blood volume<br>• Results interfered by UFH contamination in the sample, other coagulopathy, hypothermia and hemodilution |
| Anti-activated factor X (anti-FXa) | Plasma | 0.2–0.7 (0.3–0.7) units/mL | • Direct measurement of UFH effect of inhibition of FXa | • More amount of required blood volume<br>• Not widely available<br>• Required an experienced staff<br>• Higher cost<br>• Slower turnaround time<br>• Results interfered by increased bilirubin, triglyceride and plasma free hemoglobin |
| TEG and ROTEM | Whole blood | No definite cutoff | • POCT<br>• Measurement of whole blood clotting<br>• Global hemostatic test<br>• Ability to monitor other anticogulant | • No standardization<br>• No definite cutoff especially in children [26]<br>• Requirement to concomitantly interpret with other tests |

*POCT, point-of-care test; ROTEM, rotational thromboelastometry; TEG, thromboelastography.*

**Table 2.**
*The summary of methods for UFH monitoring with the target ranges of each methods [21, 23–25].*

of VTE in the previous reports, including central venous catheterization (CVC), immobilization more than 72 hours and oral contraceptive pill (OCP), are frequently found in pediatric patients who are admitted in the hospital especially children admitted in PICU [37]. Moreover, the incidence of VTE is more common in neonates and adolescents [39], hence, most VTE prophylaxis study protocols were mainly included children admitted in PICU and adolescents to prevent VTE in risky patients.

Recently Jaffrey et al. reported the new score to assess the risk of VTE development in hospitalized children including Braden Q mobility score, length of stay, CVC, history of congenital heart disease and autoimmune/inflammatory disorders in the risk assessment model (RAM) in 395 pediatric patients with the area under the curve (AUC) of 0.78 [40].

The methods to prevent VTE in children consist of physical methods e.g. intermittent pneumatic compression (IPC), graduated compression stockings (GCS) and devices and venous foot-pumps (VFPs) and pharmacological methods including oral and parenteral anticoagulants [36]. Even though the physical methods do not put the patients to be at risk of bleeding episodes, those could be applied realistically in larger children who usually weigh more than 40 kg [36]. Pharmacological prophylaxis is suggested for only children who have multiple risk factors of VTE [36] and this method should be balance with the bleeding risk of the patients. Children who require CVC, the heparin-bonded central venous line is suggested if it is available [41] due to no thrombosis was found in the report by.

## 3. Conclusions

Establishing the protocols for hemostatic control in children is very challenging due to the developmental hemostasis which make the adoption of adult protocols may not be the appropriate way. Since the evidences of hemostasis management protocols for children admitted in PICUs are still limited, more studies in this field should be warranted to close the knowledge gap and able to guide the better and more effective practice for pediatric patients in the future.

## Conflict of interest

The authors declare no conflict of interest.

## Author details

Rungrote Natesirinilkul
Faculty of Medicine, Chiang Mai University, Chiangmai, Thailand

*Address all correspondence to: rungrote.n@cmu.ac.th

## References

[1] Kenet G, Strauss T, Kaplinsky C, Paret G. Hemostasis and thrombosis in critically ill children. Seminars in Thrombosis and Hemostasis. 2008;**34**:451-458

[2] Revel-Vilk S, Rand ML, Israels SJ. Primary and secondary hemostasis, regulator of coagulation and fibrinolysis: Understanding the basics. In: Blanchette VS, Brandao LR, Breakey VR, Revel-Vilk S, editors. Sick Kids Handbook of Pediatric Thrombosis and Hemostasis. 2nd ed. Basel: Karger; 2017. pp. 8-16

[3] Ho KM, Pavey W. Applying the cell-based coagulation model in the management of critical bleeding. Anaesthesia and Intensive Care. 2017;**45**:166-176

[4] Yiu V, Natesirinilkul R, Brandao L. Disordered hemostasis and renal disorders. In: Geary DF, Schaefer F, editors. Pediatric Kidney Disease. 2nd ed. Berlin: Springer; 2016. pp. 799-821

[5] Monagle P, Barnes C, Ignjatovic V, Furmedge J, Newall F, Chan A, et al. Developmental haemostasis impact for clinical haemostasis laboratories. Thrombosis and Haemostasis. 2006;**95**:362-372

[6] Diab YA, Wong EC, Luban NL. Massive transfusion in children and neonates. British Journal of Haematology. 2013;**161**:15-26

[7] Evangelista ME, Gaffley M, Neff LP. Massive transfusion protocols for pediatric patients: Current perspectives. J Blood Med. 2020;**11**:163-172

[8] Acker SN, Hall B, Hill L, Partrick DA, Bensard DD. Adult-based massive transfusion protocol activation criteria do not work in children. European Journal of Pediatric Surgery. 2017;**27**:32-35

[9] Cunningham ME, Rosenfeld EH, Zhu H, Naik-Mathuria BJ, Russell RT, Vogel AM. A high ratio of plasma: RBC improves survival in massively transfused injured children. The Journal of Surgical Research. 2019;**233**:213-220

[10] Maw G, Furyk C. Pediatric massive transfusion: A systematic review. Pediatric Emergency Care. 2018;**34**:594-598

[11] Leeper CM, Yazer MH, Cladis FP, Saladino R, Triulzi DJ, Gaines BA. Use of uncrossmatched cold-stored whole blood in injured children with hemorrhagic shock. JAMA Pediatrics. 2018;**172**:491-492

[12] Morgan KM, Yazer MH, Triulzi DJ, Strotmeyer S, Gaines BA, Leeper CM. Safety profile of low-titer group O whole blood in pediatric patients with massive hemorrhage. Transfusion. 2021;**61**:S8-S14

[13] Wikkelsø A, Wetterslev J, Møller AM, Afshari A. Thromboelastography (TEG) or thromboelastometry (ROTEM) to monitor haemostatic treatment versus usual care in adults or children with bleeding. Cochrane Database of Systematic Reviews. 2016;**2016**:CD007871

[14] Eckert MJ, Wertin TM, Tyner SD, Nelson DW, Izenberg S, Martin MJ. Tranexamic acid administration to pediatric trauma patients in a combat setting: The pediatric trauma and tranexamic acid study (PED-TRAX). Journal of Trauma and Acute Care Surgery. 2014;77:852-858

[15] Roberts HR, Monroe DM, White GC. The use of recombinant factor VIIa in the

treatment of bleeding disorders. Blood. 2004;**104**:3858-3864

[16] McQuilten ZK, Crighton G, Engelbrecht S, Gotmaker R, Brunskill SJ, Murphy MF, et al. Transfusion interventions in critical bleeding requiring massive transfusion: A systematic review. Transfusion Medicine Reviews. 2015;**29**:127-137

[17] Maratta C, Potera RM, van Leeuwen G, Castillo Moya A, Raman L, Annich GM. Extracorporeal life support organization (ELSO): 2020 pediatric respiratory ELSO guideline. ASAIO Journal. 2020;**66**:975-979

[18] Brown G, Moynihan KM, Deatrick KB, Hoskote A, Sandhu HS, Aganga D, et al. Extracorporeal life support organization (ELSO): Guidelines for pediatric cardiac failure. ASAIO Journal. 2021;**67**:463-475

[19] Brogan T, Lequier L, Lorusso R, MacLaren G, Peek G. Extracorporeal Life Support: The ELSO Red Book. 5th ed. Ann Arbor, MI: Extracorporeal Life Support Organization; 2017

[20] Brandao LR, Diab Y, McCrindle BW. Bleeding and clotting in children with cardiac disease. In: Blanchette VS, Brandao LR, Breakey VR, Revel-Vilk S, editors. Sick Kids Handbook of Pediatric Thrombosis and Hemostasis. 2nd ed. Basel: Karger; 2017. pp. 236-260

[21] Chlebowski MM, Baltagi S, Carlson M, Levy JH, Spinella PC. Clinical controversies in anticoagulation monitoring and antithrombin supplementation for ECMO. Critical Care. 2020;**20**(24):19

[22] Dalton HJ, Reeder R, Garcia-Filion P, Holubkov R, Berg RA, Zuppa A, et al. Factors associated with bleeding and thrombosis in children receiving extracorporeal membrane oxygenation. American Journal of Respiratory and Critical Care Medicine. 2017;**196**:762-771

[23] Thomas J, Kostousov V, Teruya J. Bleeding and thrombotic complications in the use of extracorporeal membrane oxygenation. Seminars in Thrombosis and Hemostasis. 2018;**44**:20-29

[24] Barton R, Ignjatovic V, Monagle P. Anticoagulation during ECMO in neonatal and paediatric patients. Thrombosis Research. 2019;**173**:172-177

[25] Bembea MM, Annich G, Rycus P, Oldenburg G, Berkowitz I, Pronovost P. Variability in anticoagulation management of patients on extracorporeal membrane oxygenation: An international survey. Pediatric Critical Care Medicine. 2013;**14**:e77-e84

[26] Chitlur M, Sorensen B, Rivard GE, Young G, Ingerslev J, Othman M, et al. Standardization of thromboelastography: A report from the TEG-ROTEM working group. Haemophilia. 2011;**17**:532-537

[27] Biss T, Monagle T. Antithrombotic therapy in children. In: Blanchette VS, Brandao LR, Breakey VR, Revel-Vilk S, editors. Sick Kids Handbook of Pediatric Thrombosis and Hemostasis. 2nd ed. Basel: Karger; 2017. pp. 261-280

[28] Piacente C, Martucci G, Miceli V, Pavone G, Papeo A, Occhipinti G, et al. A narrative review of antithrombin use during veno-venous extracorporeal membrane oxygenation in adults: Rationale, current use, effects on anticoagulation, and outcomes. Perfusion. 2020;**35**:452-464

[29] Di Nisio M, Middeldorp S, Büller HR. Direct thrombin inhibitors. The New England Journal of Medicine. 2005;**353**:1028-1040

[30] Nagle EL, Dager WE, Duby JJ, et al. Bivalirudin in pediatric patients maintained on extracorporeal life support. Pediatric Critical Care Medicine. 2013;**14**(04):e182-e188

[31] Raffini L, Huang YS, Witmer C, Feudtner C. Dramatic increase in venous thromboembolism in children's hospitals in the United States from 2001 to 2007. Pediatrics. 2009;**124**:1001-1008

[32] Takemoto CM, Sohi S, Desai K, Bharaj R, Khanna A, McFarland S, et al. Hospital-associated venous thromboembolism in children: Incidence and clinical characteristics. The Journal of Pediatrics. 2014;**164**:332-338

[33] Choi HS, Choi CW, Kim HM, Park HW. Venous thromboembolism in pediatric patients: A single institution experience in Korea. Blood Res. 2016;**51**:164-170

[34] Schünemann HJ, Cushman M, Burnett AE, Kahn SR, Beyer-Westendorf J, Spencer FA, et al. American Society of Hematology 2018 guidelines for management of venous thromboembolism: Prophylaxis for hospitalized and nonhospitalized medical patients. Blood Advances. 2018;**2**:3198-3225

[35] Liew NC, Alemany GV, Angchaisuksiri P, Bang SM, Choi G, DE Silva DA, et al. Asian venous thromboembolism guidelines: Updated recommendations for the prevention of venous thromboembolism. International Angiology 2017;36:1-20

[36] Chalmers E, Ganesen V, Liesner R, Maroo S, Nokes T, Saunders D, et al. Guideline on the investigation, management and prevention of venous thrombosis in children. British Journal of Haematology. 2011;**154**:196-207

[37] Faustino EV, Raffini LJ. Prevention of hospital-acquired venous thromboembolism in children: A review of published guidelines. Frontiers in Pediatrics. 2017;**5**:9

[38] Monagle P, Chan AKC, Goldenberg NA, Ichord RN, Journeycake JM, Nowak-Göttl U, et al. Antithrombotic therapy in neonates and children: Antithrombotic therapy and prevention of thrombosis, 9th ed: American College of Chest Physicians Evidence-Based Clinical Practice Guidelines. Chest. 2012;**141**:e737S-e801S

[39] Andrew M, David M, Adams M, Ali K, Anderson R, Barnard D, et al. Venous thromboembolic complications (VTE) in children: First analyses of the Canadian registry of VTE. Blood. 1994;**83**:1251-1257

[40] Jaffray J, Mahajerin A, Branchford B, Nguyen ATH, Faustino EVS, Silvey M, et al. A new risk assessment model for hospital-acquired venous thromboembolism in critically ill children: A report from the Children's hospital-acquired thrombosis consortium. Pediatric Critical Care Medicine. 2022;**23**:e1-e9

[41] Pierce CM, Wade A, Mok Q. Heparin-bonded central venous lines reduce thrombotic and infective complications in critically ill children. Intensive Care Medicine. 2000;**26**:967-972

Chapter 7

# Delirium in Children after Cardiac Surgery: Brain Resuscitation

*Evgeny V. Grigoriev and Artem A. Ivkin*

## Abstract

This chapter presents the current data on delirium in children in the postoperative period with the correction of congenital heart defects. The analysis of the causes of delirium, according to the literature data, pathophysiology, clinical signs, and methods of diagnosis of postoperative delirium, is shown. In addition, methods for the prevention of delirium in children during cardiac surgery are presented.

**Keywords:** postoperative delirium, children, cardiac surgery, cardiopulmonary bypass

## 1. Introduction

Today, the problem of postoperative delirium (POD) in children is rapidly gaining relevance along with the increase in the number of anesthetic treatments in the world. Preparations for general anesthesia are constantly being improved, new, safer types appear, and outdated ones are losing popularity. The properties of all anesthetics currently used in medicine are being continuously studied. However, based on the mechanism of their action, there is no need to wait for complete safety for the brain, since the purpose of any anesthetic is to influence the functional activity of brain neurons. For children, this effect on the brain is especially dangerous. This is due to the fact that, at the age of up to 1 year, there is active development and change in the structure of the child's brain. First, an excess part of neuroblasts undergo apoptosis, and the rest of them must form dendrites and axons of neurons. Secondly, there is a process of neuronal differentiation and synaptogenesis, which underlies the cognitive development of the child. The effect of anesthetics can disrupt the fine mechanisms of regulation of the described processes and lead to impairments in the cognitive sphere in the immediate or late postoperative period [1–3]. In children, the clinical manifestation of such disorders is primarily postoperative cognitive dysfunction (POCD) and POD. POCD occurs noticeably more often—up to 80% (and even up to 100% in patients with ketamine anesthesia) [4] compared to POD, which occurs in 27–50% of patients [5, 6]. However, identifying POCD is a laborious process. Based on the classic definition given by L.S. Rasmussen et al. back in 2001, this is a cognitive disorder that develops in the early and persists in the late postoperative periods, clinically manifested in the form of impaired memory and other higher cortical functions (thinking, speech, etc.), confirmed by neuropsychological testing data in the form of a decrease in indicators testing in the postoperative period by at least 10% of the preoperative level [7]. In the realities of surgical practice, preoperative neuropsychological testing of children, despite the battery of tests available for almost all age groups, is extremely rare. This fact sharply reduces the frequency of detection of POCD in pediatric patients.

## 2. Delirium

The issue of the development of POD in children is completely different. Due to the pronounced clinical picture and the absence of the need for preoperative testing, the detection of this complication is much easier compared to POCD. Moreover, according to the studies of N. Sikich and J. Lerman, AML in children in most cases proceeds in an active form with severe symptoms [8]. This distinguishes it from POD in adults, in which up to 75% are hypoactive and mixed, and therefore hidden from diagnosis, forms, which is confirmed by their detectability, which is only 40% [9].

The current definitions of POD are presented in the Diagnostic and Statistical Manual of Mental Disorders, Fifth Edition (DSM-5) [10] and the International Statistical Classification of Diseases and Related Health Problems (ICD-10) [11], according to which the definition of POD sounds like "acute emerging disorder of consciousness with impairment of the functions of attention and understanding." The timing of its occurrence is limited to 5 days of the postoperative period. Previously, delirium was perceived not as a separate syndrome, but as an inevitable symptom, necessarily accompanying a critical state. In the literature, one can find various terms regarding POD, such as critical illness encephalopathy or ICU psychosis [12, 13]. However, for several years now, the term "postoperative delirium" has been approved, and the European Society of Anesthesiologists (ESA) even released a guideline on this condition [9], so this is the term we will use. Of particular value to us is the presence in this manual of a section devoted to the peculiarities of AML in children, even though the definition of delirium in childhood is not given there. After all, neither the DSM-5 nor the ICD-10 contains the child population. Nevertheless, this was an important step in the study of delirium in children, given that there have always been difficulties in the study of delirium in the pediatric population.

The widespread and systematic introduction of protocols for screening patients for delirium in the intensive care and intensive care units made it possible to study this issue in detail in the adult population and identify its absolute relevance. High numbers of delirium prevalence were obtained, as well as many consequences of delirium for the patient and medical organizations were revealed: dementia persisting for up to 15 months after surgery and more [14], increased mortality and morbidity in the immediate and late postoperative periods, prolongation of the period of stay patient in intensive care units, the development of dependence on the ventilator and an even higher probability of infectious complications, although the mechanism of the relationship between these complications and cognitive impairments has not yet been elucidated [15, 16]. Thus, the studied characteristics of delirium in the adult population stimulated researchers to study POD in children. However, such works are still few in number, and it is very difficult to carry out them and obtain objective data. Very revealing is a study that surveyed pediatric intensive care and intensive care units around the world about whether they routinely screen for delirium? And 75% of the respondents answered that they do not use it [17]. This is due, of course, not so much to the reluctance to carry out such screening, as the difficulties in its implementation. There is always a difference in the cognitive status, psychomotor and psycho-speech development, characteristics for each age period of the child [18, 19]. We must not forget that many diseases significantly affect the preoperative cognitive abilities of children, as happens in children with congenital heart disease (CHD). And then their cognitive potential can be strikingly different due to the variability of cerebral perfusion and oxygenation, starting from birth [20]. This implies the need for a large number of different test systems for screening for delirium. The number of scientific works devoted to the pediatric population, especially in the last 10 years, has increased dramatically, according to how the delirium assessment scales in children appear and are validated, which are clearly insufficient [21]. In recent years, data on the epidemiology and clinical features of POD in children are only beginning to accumulate.

Based on the data that are found in the world literature, the prevalence of POD in children can be represented only in the range from 2 to 80% [22–24]. The breadth of this range can be explained by the fact that research on delirium in children is carried out in different age groups, with various pathologies and types of surgical correction, so there is no one average indicator and cannot be. Against this background, it seems interesting that a large study in 2003 with the participation of 521 children, demonstrating the frequency of occurrence of delirium in different areas of surgery [25]. So, the leading position was taken by otorhinolaryngology with an indicator of 26%. At the same time, urology and orthopedics have more modest figures—15%, and abdominal surgery—13%. Quite strange data, given the absolutely different volumes of surgical intervention in the presented surgical profiles, but the authors of the article themselves could not explain this dependence. This study did not affect young patients with CHD after their surgical correction. There are two explanations for this: firstly, surgery to correct CHD is most often carried out in conditions of artificial circulation, which immediately presupposes a large set of pathological factors, which we will discuss later. Secondly, all congenital heart diseases differ greatly in their hemodynamics and, consequently, in the level of hypoxemia and blood supply to the brain, which affects the child's cognitive abilities both before and after surgery [20]. However, there are works on a group of pediatric patients undergoing cardiac surgery. For example, a study by A. Patel et al. Deserves attention, in which patients were observed from birth to 21 years after correction of various CHD [26]. Based on its results, the frequency of POD development was revealed—49%. Interestingly, in addition to the prevalence of delirium, it also revealed an increase in the number of bed days for such patients in intensive care, which coincides with the adult population. Additionally, the risk factors for the development of POD in children after this type of surgery were also considered, but this will be discussed a little later. The only drawback of this study was that it included children with a RACHS score (scale for assessing the severity and risk of CHD correction) from 1 to 6 points. In other words, a mixed assessment was carried out for all children with a wide variety of hemodynamic and cerebral oxygenation options, which, of course, cannot but affect the results [20]. Similar data are available in another study of a cohort of patients with the same type of surgery, after which the incidence of delirium was 57% [27]. Thus, the world literature does not provide data on the assessment of children with a ranking by the types of CHD and their correction, which indicates the prospects of studying this issue.

## 3. Source of problems

The best defense is an attack, and in our case, the best fight against delirium is to prevent the factors that lead to it. Many studies do not ignore these factors. Among them, one can single out those that are relevant for any surgical interventions, and those that are found only in cardiac surgery. The first group of factors is very diverse, and it is interesting that they exist even before the start of the operation. Among them, there are obvious ones, such as the administration of anticholinergic drugs or benzodiazepines for the purpose of premedication, which has long become by no means a positive tradition for many medical institutions [28, 29]. A less obvious factor that is rarely paid attention to is the increased level of preoperative anxiety in the child, which significantly increases the risk of developing POD in the postoperative period [30, 31]. If we talk about the characteristic features of children in the older age group, then it makes sense to single out the social predictors of POD: this is the male gender and the low level of education. It is also known that belonging to the white race reduces the likelihood of AML [32]. Age plays an important role in the pathophysiology of POD development. It's all about the active transformation of the child's brain—the development of neurons and interneuronal connections at the age of up to 1 year. That is why most researchers consider this age to be the most dangerous for operations in terms of the development of cognitive impairment [1–3], although there are studies on the basis of which the FDA recommends extending this age interval to 3 years. According to the same recommendations, the duration of anesthesia over 3 h is associated with an increased risk of developing POD [33]. The frequency of anesthesia, of course, also has a negative impact [34]. Regarding the anesthetic management itself, it must be remembered that inadequate analgesia can lead to the appearance of delirium, and pain is important not only from the surgery itself but also from concomitant manipulations, such as tracheal intubation or placement of a central venous catheter [9, 35, 36]. Given that the brain is a finely organized structure with special needs, metabolic imbalances in the body, such as episodes of intraoperative hypoxia or hypoglycemia at any time of the operation, are also a risk factor for the development of POD [37]. Often, such hypoxia can occur due to blood loss and acute anemia (which is very typical for cardiac surgery), in which case transfusion of erythrocyte mass and fresh frozen plasma is used. But, as recent studies show, such correction may increase the risk of postoperative cognitive impairment. The reason for this is the systemic inflammatory response (SIR) [38, 39], and we will return to it later.

More narrowly specialized is a group of factors in cardiac surgery. Such interventions are often accompanied by hemodynamic changes and infusion of sympathomimetic drugs, which is especially typical for surgical interventions in children with CHD and adversely affects cerebral perfusion and, consequently, the child's cognitive status [40, 41]. However, the widest range of factors provoking the development of postoperative cognitive disorders is cardiopulmonary bypass [42]. This is the contact of the patient's blood with the surface of the circuit of the heart-lung machine, initiating SIR [43], hemolysis due to mechanical injury of erythrocytes from the operation of roller pumps, and contact of blood with the air [44], hemodilution, which causes a decrease in the patient's hematocrit and oncotic blood pressure [26, 45]. The consequence of hemodilution and hemolysis, and not only large blood loss, explains such a frequent need for transfusion during cardiac surgery. The components of donor blood, carrying foreign material for the body, always incline it to the progression of SIR, affecting the brain [38, 46]. In a recent study, it was found that children who received at least one transfusion were twice as likely to develop POD as compared to children without a history of transfusions. Moreover, the following relationship was observed: every 10 ml of RBC transfusion per kilogram of body weight increased the likelihood of developing delirium by 90% [39].

With the introduction of the latest devices for registering microemboli in the circuit of the heart-lung machine, the problem of their influence on the cerebral vessels and cerebral ischemia that occurs, in this case, has gained relevance [47, 48]. Changes in the patient's blood temperature during cardiopulmonary bypass are also directly related to it. The whole point is in mixing the venous blood flowing into the cardiotomy reservoir (the temperature of which is always lower) and the arterial blood flowing out of the oxygenator (most often having a temperature that is familiar to humans—about 37°C). With this mixing, air bubbles are formed from the liquid part of the blood, which can get to the patient, causing air microembolism [49]. Temperature control is also important to avoid cerebral hyperthermia, which can negatively affect the brain [50].

Of great importance is not only the fact of cardiopulmonary bypass but also its duration, as well as the time of clamping of the aorta (actually ischemia of the heart myocardium) [37]. All of these factors, in addition to their direct destructive effect on the brain, ultimately initiate and enhance the development of SIR [43, 51]. The combination of such a variety of factors determines the entire complex of the pathophysiology of brain damage.

However, the problem is also that the onset of delirium is influenced not only by intraoperative but also by many factors of the immediate postoperative period. For cardiac surgery (especially in children), this period is always difficult due to the volume of interventions. Often, a long stay in the intensive care unit is required, due to which patients experience stress caused by medical manipulations, noise and disturbance of circadian rhythms, pain syndrome, and many other factors [52, 53]. In an attempt to neutralize at least some of these factors, benzodiazepines are often used (especially in patients on mechanical ventilation). But such an aspiration does not always benefit the patient and, based on recent studies, increases not only the incidence of POD, but also the length of stay in the intensive care unit [54, 55]. It is also interesting that the harmful effect of benzodiazepines can be enhanced by the administration of anticholinergic drugs [56]. Often, patients require prolonged mechanical ventilation, which is directly related to the risk of delirium. A recent study shows that any form of respiratory support can lead to the development of delirium. Of course, invasive artificial ventilation of the lungs with the presence of an endotracheal tube in a child has the greatest effect on him; nevertheless, attention is drawn to the fact that even the use of nasal cannulas for oxygen therapy can increase the risk of developing AML [26].

## 4. A bit of pathophysiology and clarity

The brain has a special type of structure and interaction of cells, and SIR (which was given great attention in the previous section) manifests itself in it as a neuroinflammatory response, which determines all the disorders that are clinically manifested in a patient [57]. If we want to understand the essence of this process, then we need to look at the theory of the neurovascular unit of the brain (NVU).

The fact is that regulatory processes in the brain are a special type of cell interaction that requires the creation of an isolated microenvironment. For this purpose, there is the blood-brain barrier (BBB) and its components, the functional unit of which is NVU. NVU consists of microvessels that are associated with astrocytes, which in turn are associated with neurons and their axons. The BBB contains special carrier proteins for the selective transport of substances from blood plasma to neurons. All this in combination ensures the coordinated work of the brain through intercellular communications and metabolic coupling of cells of the central nervous system [58]. Cerebral injury leads to the activation of microglia and astrocytes and the sequential production of inflammatory mediators in the brain [59]. Mediators damage the BBB and further stimulate cell death and gliosis [60]. Moreover, when the integrity of the BBB is violated, the NVU can be influenced not only by local but also by systemic cytokines (recall the notorious SIR). They stimulate the expression of adhesion molecules, potentiate the adhesion and extravasation of neutrophils and monocytes into ischemic tissues [61]. Local production of chemokines enhances leukocyte extravasation in these tissues [62]. All of these processes occur within the NVU, producing certain pathological changes in the tissues of the brain, followed by its dysfunction. Summarizing the above, we can conclude that not only destructive factors such as hypoxia have a damaging effect on the brain, but also any other factors that can cause SIR [63, 64]. In addition, one should not forget about the physiological features of children, because the first year of life in them is characterized by increased permeability of the vascular wall and hydrophilicity of the interstitial space, which, of course, further contributes to the accumulation of excess fluid in it and increased SIR [65].

As you may have noticed, almost all etiological factors realized by such complex pathophysiological mechanisms are modifiable, and they can and should be combated! However, in some cases, even after making every effort, you will still encounter delirium after the operation. But you still need to be able to recognize it.

## 5. You need to know the enemy by sight, or how not to pass by delirium

Aggression, sometimes with self-damaging actions (attempts to remove drainage tubes, venous catheters, etc.), agitation, insomnia, disturbance of circadian rhythms, depression, disorientation, uncontrolled speech, short-term memory disturbances, hallucinations, impaired perception, decreased attention level, disturbances consciousness [66]. All this is a description of various manifestations of POD in children. Of course, there is nothing new in it, and almost every doctor who works with children in the postoperative period has encountered such manifestations. The question is: how to distinguish such a clinical picture from the normal behavior of a child who is simply experiencing a feeling of fear and anxiety and wants to be close to his parents as soon as possible? Special scales come to the rescue. There are not so many of them in pediatric practice, but they all have a high diagnostic value. And this value rises sharply in the field of cardiac surgery. First of all, this is due to the fact that most children after cardiac surgery are in the intensive care unit and intensive care, and contact with them is often difficult due to prolonged mechanical ventilation and the presence of an endotracheal tube or tracheostomy cannula. However, in modern scales, such difficulties are taken into account, as are the characteristics of children of all ages [67]. Let us consider a few of them.

As described earlier, POD in children is most often found in a hyperactive form with severe symptoms [8]. Such delirium is commonly referred to in international guidelines as emergence delirium [68]. In this case, it is necessary to carry out a differential diagnosis between the child's agitation after surgery and this type of delirium. Agitation is characterized by anxiety and discomfort in the child. Emergence delirium includes a wider range of symptoms: disorders of the child's consciousness, in particular, disorientation in the outside world, changes in perception, including hypersensitivity to stimuli, and the appearance of hyperactive motor skills during awakening from anesthesia with no success in trying to calm the child [69, 70]. It is easier to carry out such differential diagnosis using The Pediatric Anesthesia Emergence Delirium (PAED) scale. The assessment is carried out quickly, in 5 blocks: the child's eye contact with others, the purposefulness of his actions, his ability to become aware of his surroundings, the general level of anxiety, and the child's reaction to attempts to calm him down. Points are assigned from 0 to 4 for each block [8]. The maximum total score is 20. The result of 10 points or more indicates the presence of emergence delirium with a sensitivity level of 64% and a specificity of 86%, 12 points or more—100% and 94.5%, respectively [71]. Such a high level of sensitivity can be explained by the specialization of the scale specifically from the emergence of delirium with severe symptoms. If we are talking about using it to diagnose all types of delirium, then its sensitivity is not yet clear enough and, according to some researchers, does not exceed 50% [72].

PAED, as already noted, has a very low sensitivity to hypoactive forms of delirium, and a different scale is required for their detection. This role can be played by The Cornell Assessment for Pediatric Delirium (CAPD), which is, in fact, a modified PAED scale (see **Table 1**). The changes consist of the addition of three new assessment units to those already existing in PAED, and they are aimed precisely at the detection of the hypoactive form of delirium [73]. The following areas of assessment have emerged: the need for communication, inadequate level of activity while awake, and delayed response when interacting with the child. Similarly, a score for each block is given from 0 to 4 points, and a result of 9 points or more indicates the presence of POD. Studies showing different levels of sensitivity and specificity depending on the age of the patient cannot be ignored. So, for example, for children over 13 years of age, the specificity is 98%, but the sensitivity reaches only 50%. The situation is mirrored in the group of children under 2 years of age, in which the specificity will already be only 68%, but the sensitivity will be 100% [74, 75]. As for the age at which to start using the PAED and CAPD scales, most studies agree at the age of 1.5 years. The presented scales are a good example of the fact that the assessment of AML in the

| **Criteria** | **Never**<br>**4** | **Rarely**<br>**3** | **Sometimes**<br>**2** | **Often**<br>**1** | **Always**<br>**0** | **Score** |
|---|---|---|---|---|---|---|
| Does the child make eye contact with the caregiver? | | | | | | |
| Are the child's actions purposeful? | | | | | | |
| Is the child aware of his/her surroundings? | | | | | | |
| Does the child communicate needs and wants? | | | | | | |
| | Never<br>0 | Rarely<br>1 | Sometimes<br>2 | Often<br>3 | Always<br>4 | |
| The child is restless | | | | | | |
| Is the child inconsolable? | | | | | | |
| Is the child underactive very little movement while awake? | | | | | | |
| Does it take the child a long time to respond to interactions? | | | | | | |
| Total score | | | | | | |

**Table 1.**
*Cornell assessment of pediatric delirium scale [73].*

| | |
|---|---|
| Ultrafiltration [78, 79] | Maintaining colloidal-oncotic blood pressure by removing excess fluid. An additional effect is the elimination of inflammatory mediators in the composition of the ultrafiltrate |
| Filtration of the primary filling volume before the start of cardiopulmonary bypass [43] | Removal of various foreign particles that were formed during the assembly of the artificial circulation circuit and can provoke the development of a systemic inflammatory response |
| Leukocyte filter [80] | A decrease in the number of leukocytes and, as a consequence, a weakening of the reaction of systemic inflammation. Both the patient's own leukocytes and those in transfusion media can be removed |
| Various technical perfusion solutions (minimization of the cardiopulmonary bypass circuit, biocompatible circuits, limiting the work of cardiotomy aspirators, minimizing the prime) [81–83] | The use of these methods leads to a decrease in the secretion of various proinflammatory cytokines, a weakening of the activation of complement and leukocytes in comparison with the conventional circuitry. There is a significant decrease in red blood cell damage, activation of coagulation cascades, fibrinolytic and pro-inflammatory activity |
| Aprotinin [84] | Aprotinin inhibits a receptor (protease-activated receptors) expressed on the surface of platelets and endothelial cells, leading to blocking the aggregation process and reducing inflammation |
| Glucocorticoids [85, 86] | For example, methylprednisolone at a dose of 30 mg per 1 kg of body weight, according to studies, reduces the production of IL-6 and IL-8, but not IL-10 and IL-1ra. These results indicate that one of the mechanisms of the cytoprotective action of methylprednisolone may be the effect on the pro-inflammatory and anti-inflammatory cytokine balance. It should be noted that the effect of systemic glucocorticoids on the development of infection in the postoperative period |
| Hypothermia [87–89] | Based on the data of modern studies of the use of hypothermia in pediatric cardiac surgery, it can be said that it effectively reduces the metabolic rate, but does not contribute to the proper extent to the prevention or decrease in the severity of the systemic inflammatory response |

**Table 2.**
*Prevention and relief of systemic inflammatory response [43, 78–89].*

conditions of the intensive care unit does not take much time and effort, but it can bring a lot of new information about the patient. It is only important to do it regularly and, of course, only after assessing the child on a pain scale convenient for a doctor, for example, FLACC, NIPS, or Wong-Baker [76].

There are many works on the effect of POD on clinical outcomes and on the undoubted increase in the duration of hospitalization and even mortality [24]. The question of the impact of POD on the cognitive development of a child in the long term is also important. How much is it possible to compensate for the resulting damage to the brain and further return to normal indicators of its performance? Such questions are just beginning to be investigated and do not yet have a sufficient evidence base [77].

As mentioned above, SIR and neuroinflammation play an important role in the formation of cerebral damage. In the conditions of modern anesthetic technology and perfusion, a considerable amount of information has accumulated on various methods of preventing SIR, which are effective to a greater or lesser extent. We offer an overview of the most commonly used methods for the prevention of SIR (see **Table 2**) [43, 78–89].

Apparently, the future in POD treatment and prevention lies with complex strategies. Even though new drugs are constantly being developed and studies are being carried out on those that have long been used in practice, they will never be able to compare their safety with non-pharmacological measures of influence on the child. Creation in the perioperative period of a calm psycho-emotional environment, as close as possible to a comfortable one for the child, is, along with the elimination of all provoking factors, the key to the prevention of postoperative delirium. An increasing number of researchers are coming to such conclusions. It turns out that even such a simple therapeutic method as massage in the postoperative period can help in the fight against POD [90]. Of course, complex methods of prevention and treatment of delirium are immeasurably more effective. An example is the ADVANCE strategy presented in the above-mentioned ESA guideline [9]. It is interesting that it offers not only the traditional work of the medical staff with the child but also the use of various interactive technologies with the active participation of parents, which is of paramount importance for young patients.

## Author details

Evgeny V. Grigoriev[1] and Artem A. Ivkin[2]*

1 Anesthesiology and Intensive Care Department, Deputy Director for Research and Therapy, Kuzbass Cardiology Center, Kemerovo Region, Russia

2 Kuzbass Cardiology Center, Kemerovo, Russian Federation

*Address all correspondence to: aai-tema@mail.ru

## References

[1] Hansen TG. Anesthesia-related neurotoxicity and the developing animal brain is not a significant problem in children. Paediatric Anaesthesia. 2015;**25**(1):65-72. DOI: 10.1111/pan.12548

[2] Jevtovic-Todorovic V. General anesthetics and neurotoxicity: How much do we know? Anesthesiology Clinics. 2016;**34**(3):439-451. DOI: 10.1016/j.anclin.2016.0 4.001

[3] Lesny I. Developmental disorders of the central nervous system. Developmental Medicine and Child Neurology. 1960;**2**(2):103. DOI: 10.1111/j.1469-8749.1960.tb05151.x

[4] Ovezov AM, Lobov MA, Panteleeva MV, Lugovoy AV, Myatchin PS, Guskov IE. Correction of early cognitive impairment in school-age children operated on under conditions of total intravenous anesthesia. Anesthesiology and Reanimatology. 2012;**3**:25-29

[5] Meyburg J, Dill ML, Traube C, Silver G, von Haken R. Patterns of post-operative delirium in children. Pediatric Critical Care Medicine. 2017;**18**(2): 128-133. DOI: 10.1097/PCC.0000000000000993

[6] Cho EA, Cha YB, Shim JG, Ahn JH, Lee SH, Ryu KH. Comparison of single minimum dose administration of dexmedetomidine and midazolam for prevention of emergence delirium in children: A randomized controlled trial. Journal of Anesthesia. 2020;**34**(1):59-65. DOI: 10.1007/s00540-019-02705-6

[7] Rasmussen LS, Larsen K, Houx P, Skovgaard LT, Hanning CD, Moller JT, et al. The assessment of postoperative cognitive function. Acta Anaesthesiologica Scandinavica. 2001;**45**(3):275-289. DOI: 10.1034/j.1399-6576.2001.0 45003275

[8] Sikich N, Lerman J. Development and psychometric evaluation of the pediatric anesthesia emergence delirium scale. Anesthesiology. 2004;**100**(5):1138-1145. DOI: 10.1097/00000542-200 405000-00015

[9] Aldecoa C, Bettelli G, Bilotta F, Sanders RD, Audisio R, Borozdina A, et al. European Society of Anaesthesiology evidence-based and consensus-based guidelines on postoperative delirium. European Journal of Anaesthesiology. 2017;**34**(4):192-214. DOI: 10.1097/EJA.0000000000000594

[10] American Psychiatric Association. Diagnostic and statistical manual of mental disorders (Dsm-51). 5th ed. Amer. Psychiatric Pub. Inc.; 2013. Available from: https://www.academia.edu/32447322/DIAGNOSTIC_AND_STATISTI-CAL_MANUAL_OF_MENTAL_DISORDERS. [Accessed: November 18, 2020]

[11] International Statistical Classification of Diseases and Related Health Problems. 10th Revision. Available from: https://icd.who.int/browse10/2016/en [Accessed: November 08, 2020]

[12] Ely EW, Margolin R, Francis J, May L, Truman B, Dittus R, et al. Evaluation of delirium in critically ill patients: Validation of the confusion assessment method for the intensive care unit (CAM-ICU). Critical Care Medicine. 2001;**29**(7):1370-1379. DOI:10.1097/00003246-200107000-00012

[13] Justic M. Does "ICU psychosis" really exist? Critical Care Nurse.

2000;**20**(3):28-37; quiz 38-29. DOI: 10.4037/ccn2000.20.3.28

[14] Sprung J, Roberts RO, Weingarten TN, Cavalcante AN, Knopman DS, Petersen RC, et al. Postoperative delirium in elderly patients is associated with subsequente cognitive impairment. British Journal of Anaesthesia. 2017;**119**(2):316-323. DOI: 10.1093/bja/aex130

[15] Gottesman RF, Grega MA, Bailey MM, Pham LD, Zeger SL, Baumgartner WA, et al. Delirium after coronary artery bypass graft surgery and late mortality. Annals of Neurology. 2010;**67**(3):338-344. DOI: 10.1002/ana.21899

[16] Brown C, Laflam A, Max L, Lymar D, Neufeld KJ, Tian J, et al. The impact of delirium after cardiac surgical procedures on postoperative resource use. Annals of Thoracic Surgery. 2016;**101**(5):1663-1669. DOI: 10.1016/j.athoracsur.2015.12.074

[17] Staveski SL, Pickler RH, Lin L, Shaw RJ, Meinzen-Derr J, Redington A, et al. Management of pediatric delirium in pediatric cardiac intensive care patients: An international survey of current practices. Pediatric Critical Care Medicine. 2018;**19**(6):538-543. DOI: 10.1097/PCC.0000000000001558

[18] Smith HA, Gangopadhyay M, Goben CM, Jacobowski NL, Chestnut MH, Savage S, et al. The preschool confusion assessment method for the ICU: Valid and reliable delirium monitoring for critically ill infants and children. Critical Care Medicine. 2016;**44**(3):592-600. DOI: 10.1097/ccm.0000000000001428

[19] Schieveld JN, Leroy PL, van Os J, Nicolai J, Vos GD, Leentjens AF. Pediatric delirium in critical illness: Phenomenology, clinical correlates and treatment response in 40 cases in the pediatric intensive care unit. Intensive Care Medicine. 2007;**33**(6):1033-1040. DOI: 10.1007/s00134-007-0637-8

[20] Calderon J, Bellinger DC. Executive function deficits in congenital heart disease: Why is intervention important? Cardiology in the Young. 2015;**25**(7):1238-1246. DOI: 10.1017/S1047951115001134

[21] Walker T, Kudchadkar SR. Pain and sedation management: 2018 update for the Rogers' text-book of pediatric intensive care. Pediatric Critical Care Medicine. 2019;**20**(1):54-61. DOI: 10.1097/pcc.0000000000001765

[22] Dervan LA, Di Gennaro JL, Farris RWD, Watson RS. Delirium in a Tertiary PICU. Pediatric Critical Care Medicine. 2020;**21**(1):21-32. DOI: 10.1097/pcc.0000000000002126

[23] Ali I, Alahdal M, Xia H, El Moughrabi S, A, Shiqian H, Yao S. Ketofol performance to reduce postoperative emergence agitation in children undergoing adenotonsillectomy. The Libyan Journal of Medicine. 2020;**15**(1):1688450. DOI: 10.1080/19932820.2019.1688450

[24] Traube C, Silver G, Gerber LM, Kaur S, Mauer EA, Kerson A, et al. Delirium and mortality in critically ill children: Epidemiology and outcomes of pediatric delirium. Critical Care Medicine. 2017;**45**(5):891-898. DOI: 10.1097/CCM.0000000000002324

[25] Voepel-Lewis T, Malviya S, Tait AR. A prospective cohort study of emergence agitation in the pediatric postanesthesia care unit. Anesthesia and Analgesia. 2003;**96**(6):1625-1630. DOI: 10.1213/01.ane.00000 62522.210 48.61

[26] Patel AK, Biagas KV, Clarke EC. Delirium in children after cardiac bypass surgery. Pediatric Critical Care Medicine.

2017;**18**(2):165-171. DOI: 10.1097/PCC.0000000000001032

[27] Alvarez RV, Palmer C, Czaja AS, Peyton C, Silver G, Traube MPM, et al. Delirium is a common and early finding in patients in the pediatric cardiac intensive care unit. The Journal of Pediatrics. 2018;**195**:206-212. DOI: 10.1016/j.jpeds.2017.11.064

[28] Federico A, Tamburin S, Maier A, Faccini M, Casari R, Morbioli L, et al. Multifocal cognitive dysfunction in high-dose benzodiazepine users: A cross-sectional study. Neurology Science. 2017;**3**(1):137-142. DOI: 10.1007/s10072-016-2732-5

[29] Hughes CG, Pandharipande PP, Ely EW. Delirium. Springer; 2020. DOI: 10.1007/978-3-030-25751-4

[30] Beringer RM, Segar P, Pearson A, Greamspet M, Kilpatrick N. Observational study of perioperative behavior changes in children having teeth extracted under general anesthesia. Paediatric Anaesthesia. 2014;**24**(5):499-504. DOI: 10.1111/pan.12362

[31] Kühlmann A, Lahdo N, Lonneke M, van Dijk SM. What are the validity and reliability of the modified Yale preoperative anxiety scale-short form in children less than 2 years old? Pediatric Anesthesia. 2018;**29**(2):137-143. DOI: 10.1111/pan.13536

[32] Rudolph JL, Jones RN, Levkoff SE, Rockett C, Inouye SK, Sellke FW, et al. Derivation and validation of a preoperative prediction rule for delirium after cardiac surgery. Circulation. 2009;**119**(2):229-236. DOI: 10.1161/CIRCULATIONAHA.108.795260

[33] United States Food and Drug Administration. FDA Drug Safety Communication: FDA Review Results in New Warnings about Using General Anesthetics and Sedation Drugs in Young Children and Pregnant Women. 2016. Available from: https://www.fda.gov/drugs/drug-safety-and-availability/fda-drug-safety-communication-fda-review-results-new-warnings-about-using-general-an-esthetics [Accessed: November 18, 2020]

[34] Shi Y, Hu D, Rodgers EL, Katusic SK, Gleich SJ, Hanson AC, et al. Epidemiology of general anesthesia prior to age 3 in a population-based birth cohort. Paediatric Anaesthesia. 2018;**28**(6):513-519. DOI: 10.1111/pan.13359

[35] Dahmani S, Stany I, Brasher C, Lejeune C, Bruneau B, Wood C, et al. Pharmacological prevention of sevoflurane- and desflurane-related emergence agitation in children: A meta-analysis of published studies. British Journal of Anaesthesia. 2010;**104**:216-223. DOI: 10.1093/bja/aep376

[36] Pickard A, Davies P, Birnie K, Beringer R. Systematic review and meta-analysis of the effect of intraoperative α2-adrenergic agonists on postoperative behaviour in children. British Journal of Anaesthesia. 2014;**112**:982-990. DOI: 10.1093/bja/aeu093

[37] Kazmierski J, Kowman M, Banach M, Fendler W, Okonski P, Banys A, et al. Incidence and predictors of delirium after cardiac surgery: Results from the IPDACS study. Journal of Psychosomatic Research. 2010;**69**(2):179-185. DOI: 10.1016/j.jpsychores.2010.02.009

[38] Delaney M, Stark PC, Suh M, Triulzi DJ, Hess JR, Steiner ME, et al. The impact of blood component ratios on clinical outcomes and survival. Anesthesia and Analgesia. 2017;**124**(6):1777-1782. DOI: 10.1213/ANE.0000000000001926

[39] Nellis ME, Goel R, Feinstein S, Shahbaz S, Kaur S, Traube C. Association between transfusion of RBCs and subsequent development of delirium in critically ill children. Pediatric Critical Care Medicine. 2018;**19**(10):925-929. DOI: 10.1097/PCC.0000000000001675

[40] Hogue CW Jr, Palin CA, Arrowsmith JE. Cardiopulmonary bypass management and neurologic outcomes: An evidence-based appraisal of current practices. Anesthesia and Analgesia. 2006;**103**(1):21-37. DOI: 10.1213/01.ane.0000220035.82989.79

[41] Hori D, Brown C, Ono M, Rappold T, Sieber F, Gottschalk A, et al. Arterial pressure above the upper cerebral autoregulation limit during cardiopulmonary bypass is associated with postoperative delirium. British Journal of Anaesthesia. 2014;**113**(6):1009-1017. DOI: 10.1093/bja/aeu319

[42] Hirata Y. Cardiopulmonary bypass for pediatric cardiac surgery. General Thoracic and Cardiovascular Surgery. 2018;**66**(2):65-70. DOI: 10.1007/s11748-017-0870-1

[43] Myers GJ, Wegner J. Endothelial glycocalyx and cardiopulmonary bypass. Journal of ExtraCorporeal Technology. 2017;**49**(3):174-181

[44] Toomasian CJ, Aiello SR, Drumright BL, Major TC, Bartlett RH, Toomasian JM. The effect of air exposure on leucocyte and cytokine activation in an in-vitro model of cardiotomy suction. Perfusion. 2018;**33**(7):538-545. DOI: 10.1177/0267659118766157

[45] Baker RA, Nikolic A, Onorati F, Alston RP. 2019 EACTS/EACTA/EBCP guidelines on cardiopulmonary bypass in in adult cardiac surgery: A tool to better clinical practice. European Journal of Cardio-Thoracic Surgery. 2020;**57**(2):207-209. DOI: 10.1093/ejcts/ezz358

[46] Ferraris VA, Ballert EQ, Mahan A. The relationship between intraoperative blood transfusion and postoperative systemic inflammatory response syndrome. The American Journal of Surgery. 2013;**205**(4):457-465. DOI: 10.1016/j.amjsurg.2012.07.0 42

[47] Stehouwer MC, Boers C, Vroege R, Kelder JC, Yilmaz A, Bruins P. Clinical evaluation of the air removal characteristics of an oxygenator with integrated arterial filter in a minimized extracorporeal circuit. The International Journal of Artificial Organs. 2011;**34**(4):374-382. DOI: 10.5301/ijao.2011.7749

[48] Reis EE, Menezes LD, Justo CCL. Gaseous microemboli in cardiac surgery with cardiopulmonary bypass: The use of veno-arterial shunts as preventive method. Evista Brasileira de Cirurgia Cardiovascular. 2012;**27**(3):436-445. DOI: 10.5935/1678-9741.20120073

[49] Engelman R, Baker RA, Likosky DS. The Society of Thoracic Surgeons, the Society of Cardiovascular Anesthesiologists, and the American Society of ExtraCorporeal Technology: Clinical practice guidelines for cardiopulmonary bypass—Temperature management during cardiopulmonary bypass. Jouranal of ExtraCorporeal Technology. 2015;**47**(3):145-154

[50] Grigore AM, Murray CF, Ramakrishna H, Djaiani G. A core review of temperature regimens and neuroprotection during cardiopulmonary bypass: Does rewarming rate matter? Anesthesia and Analgesia. 2009;**109**(6):1741-1751. DOI: 10.1213/ANE.0b013e3181c0 4fea

[51] Wang Y, Lin X, Yue H, Kissoon N, Sun B. Evaluation of systemic

inflammatory response syndrome-negative sepsis from a Chinese regional pediatric network. Collaborative Study Group for Pediatric Sepsis in Huai'an. BMC Pediatrics. 2019;**19**(1):11. DOI: 10.1186/s12887-018-1364-8

[52] Coppola S, Caccioppola A, Chiumello D. Internal clock and the surgical ICU patient. Current Opinion in Anesthesiology. 2020;**33**(2):177-184. DOI: 10.1097/ACO.0000000000000816

[53] Pandharipande P, Shintani A, Peterson J, Pun BT, Wilkinson GR, Dittus RS, et al. Lorazepam is an independent risk factor for transitioning to delirium in intensive care unit patients. Anesthesiology. 2006;**104**(1):21-26. DOI: 10.1097/00000542-200601000-00005

[54] Mody K, Kaur S, Mauer EA, Gerber LM, Greenwald BM, Silver G, et al. Benzodiazepines and development of delirium in critically ill children: Estimating the causal effect. Critical Care Medicine. 2018;**46**(9):1486-1491. DOI: 10.1097/CCM.0000000000003194

[55] Smith HAB, Gangopadhyay M, Goben CM, Jacobowski NL, Chestnut MH, Thompson JL, et al. Delirium and benzodiazepines associated with prolonged ICU stay in critically ill infants and young children. Critical Care Medicine. 2017;**45**(9):1427-1435. DOI: 10.1097/CCM.0000000000002515

[56] Madden K, Hussain K, Tasker RC. Anticholinergic medication burden in pediatric prolonged critical illness: A potentially modifiable risk factor for delirium. Pediatric Critical Care Medicine. 2018;**19**(10):917-924. DOI: 10.1097/PCC.0000000000001658

[57] Cerejeira J, Firmino H, Vazserra A, Mukaetova-Ladinska EB. The neuroinflammatory hypothesis of delirium. Acta Neuropathologica. 2010;**119**:737-754. DOI: 10.1007/s00 401-010-0 674-1

[58] Torbett BE, Baird A, Eliceiri BP. Understanding the rules of the road: Proteomic approaches to interrogate the blood brain barrier. Frontiers in Neuroscience. 2015;**9**:70. DOI: 10.3389/fnins.2015.00070

[59] Denes A, Vidyasagar R, Feng J, Narvainen J, McColl BW, Kauppinen RA, et al. Proliferating resident microglia after focal cerebral ischaemia in mice. Journal of Cerebral Blood Flow and Metabolism. 2007;**27**(12):1941-1953. DOI: 10.1038/sj.jcbfm.9600 495

[60] Kaushal V, Schlichter LC. Mechanisms of microglia-mediated neurotoxicity in a new model of the stroke penumbra. Journal of Neuroscience. 2008;**28**(9):2221-2230. DOI: 10.1523/JNEUROSCI.5643-07.2008

[61] Christov A, Ottman JT, Grammas P. Vascular inflammatory, oxidative and protease-based processes: Implications for neuronal cell death in Alzheimer's disease. Neurological Research. 2004;**26**(5):540-546. DOI: 10.1179/01616 410 4225016218

[62] Minami M, Satoh M. Chemokines and their receptors in the brain: Pathophysiological roles in ischemic brain injury. Life Sciences. 2003;**74**(2-3):321-327. DOI: 10.1016/j.lfs.2003.09.019

[63] Pozhilenkova EA, Lopatina OL, Komleva YK, Salmin VV, Salmina AB. Blood-brain barrier-supported neurogenesis in healthy and diseased brain. Nature Reviews Neuroscience. 2017;**28**(4):397-415. DOI: 10.1515/revneuro-2016-0071

[64] Salmina AB, Komleva YK, Kuvacheva NV, Lopatina OL,

Pozhilenkova EA, Gorina YV, et al. Inflammation and aging of the brain. Vestnik Rossijskoj AMN. 2015;**1**:17-25

[65] Tassani P, Schad H, Winkler C, Bernhard A, Ettner U, Braun SL, et al. Capillary leak syndrome after cardiopulmonary bypass in elective, uncomplicated coronary artery bypass grafting operations: Does it exist? The Journal of Thoracic and Cardiovascular Surgery. 2002;**123**(4):735-741. DOI: 10.1067/mtc.2002.120348

[66] Holly C, Porter S, Echevarria M, Dreker M, Ruzehaji S. CE: Original research: Recognizing delirium in hospitalized children: A systematic review of the evidence on risk factors and characteristics. The American Journal of Nursing. 2018;**118**(4):24-36. DOI: 10.1097/01.NAJ.0000532069.55339.f9

[67] Nevid JS. Essentials of Psychology: Concepts and Applications. 5th ed. Cengage Learning: Australia; 2018

[68] Coté CJ, Lerman J, Anderson BJ. A Practice of Anesthesia for Infants and Children. 6th ed. Philadelphia: Elsevier; 2019

[69] Costi D, Cyna AM, Ahmed S, Stephens K, Strickland P, Ellwood J, et al. Effects of sevoflurane versus other general anaesthesia on emergence agitation in children. The Cochrane Database of Systematic Reviews. 2014;(9):CD007084. DOI: 10.1002/14651858.CD007084.pub2

[70] Vlajkovic GP, Sindjelic RP. Emergence delirium in children: Many questions, few answers. Anesthesia and Analgesia. 2007;**104**(1):84-91. DOI: 10.1213/01.ane.0000250914.91881.a8

[71] Lerman J. Emergence delirium and agitation in children. UpToDate. 2017. Available from: https://www.uptodate.com/contents/emergence-delirium-and-agitation-in-children. [Accessed: November 08, 2020]

[72] Silver G, Traube C, Kearney J, Kelly D, Yoon MJ, Moyal WN, et al. Detecting pediatric delirium: Development of a rapid observational assessment tool. Intensive Care Medicine. 2012;**38**(6):1025-1031. DOI: 10.1007/s00134-012-2518-z

[73] Traube C, Silver G, Kearney J. Cornell assessment of pediatric delirium: A valid, rapid, observational tool for screening delirium in the PICU. Critcal Care Medicine. 2014;**42**(3):656-663. DOI: 10.1097/CCM.0b013e3182a66b76

[74] Bettencourt A, Mullen JE. Delirium in children: Identification, prevention, and management. Critical Care Nurse. 2017;**37**(3):9-18. DOI: 10.4037/ccn2017692

[75] Simone S, Edwards S, Lardieri A. Implementation of an ICU bundle: An interprofessional quality improvement project to enhance delirium management and monitor delirium prevalence in a single PICU. Pediatric Critical Care Medicine. 2017;**18**(6):531-540. DOI: 10.1097/PCC.0000000000001127

[76] Somaini M, Engelhardt T, Fumagalli R, Ingelmo PM. Emergence delirium or pain after anaesthesia—How to distinguish between the two in young children: A retrospective analysis of observational studies. British Journal of Anaesthesia. 2016;**116**(3):377-383. DOI: 10.1093/bja/aev552

[77] Meyburg J, Ries M, Zielonka M. Cognitive and behavioral consequences of pediatric delirium: A pilot study. Pediatric Critical Care Medicine. 2018;**19**(10):531-537. DOI: 10.1097/PCC.0000000000001686

[78] Chen F, You Y, Ding P, Wu K, Mo X. Effects of balanced ultrafiltration

during extracorporeal circulation for children with congenital heart disease on postoperative serum inflammatory response. Fetal and Pediatric Pathology. 2020;**39**(5):401-408. DOI: 10.1080/15513815.2019.1661050

[79] Bierer J, Stanzel R, Henderson M, Sett S, Horne D. Ultrafiltration in pediatric cardiac surgery review. World Journal for Pediatric and Congenital Heart Surgery. 2019;**10**(6):778-788. DOI: 10.1177/2150135119870176

[80] Alexiou C, Tang AA, Sheppard SV, Smith DC, Gibbs R, Livesey SA, et al. The effect of leucodepletion on leucocyte activation, pulmonary inflammation and respiratory index in surgery for coronary revascularisation: A prospective randomised study. European Journal of Cardio-Thoracic Surgery. 2004;**26**(2):294-300. DOI: 10.1016/j.ejcts.200 4.0 4.017

[81] Pereira SN, Zumba IB, Batista MS, Pieve DD, Santos ED, Stuermer R, et al. Comparison of two technics of cardiopulmonary bypass (conventional and mini CPB) in the trans- and postoperative periods of cardiac surgery. Revista Brasileira de Cirurgia Cardiovascular. 2015;**30**(4):433-442. DOI: 10.5935/1678-9741.201500 46

[82] Holmannova D, Kolackova M, Mandak J, Kunes P, Holubcova Z, Holubec T, et al. Effects of conventional CPB and mini-CPB on neutrophils CD162, CD166 and CD195 expression. Perfusion. 2017;**32**(2):141-150. DOI: 10.1177/0267659116669586

[83] Nguyen B, Luong L, Naase H, Vives M, Jakaj G, Finch J, et al. Sulforaphane pretreatment prevents systemic inflammation and renal injury in response to cardiopulmonary bypass. The Journal of Thoracic and Cardiovascular Surgery. 2014;**148**(2):690-697.e3. DOI: 10.1016/j.jtcvs.2013.12.0 48

[84] Ferreira CA, Vicente WV, Evora PR, Rodrigues AJ, Klamt JG, Carlotti AP, et al. Assessment of aprotinin in the reduction of inflammatory systemic response in children undergoing surgery with cardiopulmonary bypass. Revista Brasileira de Cirurgia Cardiovascular. 2010;**25**(1):85-98. DOI: 10.1590/s0102-76382010000100018

[85] Whitlock RP, Devereaux PJ, Teoh KH, Lamy A, Vincent J, Pogue J, et al. Methylprednisolone in patients undergoing cardiopulmonary bypass (SIRS): A randomised, double-blind, placebo-controlled trial. Lancet. 2015;**386**(10000):1243-1253. DOI: 10.1016/S0140-6736(15)00273-1

[86] Dreher M, Glatz AC, Kennedy A, Rosenthal T, Gaynor JW. A single-center analysis of methylprednisolone use during pediatric cardiopulmonary bypass. The Journal of ExtraCorporeal Technology. 2015;**47**(3):155-159

[87] Kaplan M, Karaagac A, Can T, Yilmaz S, Yesilkaya MI, Olsun A, et al. Open heart surgery at patient's own temperature without active cooling. The Heart Surgery Forum. 2018;**21**(3):132-138. DOI: 10.1532/hsf.1985

[88] Schmitt KR, Fedarava K, Justus G, Redlin M, Böttcher W, Delmo Walter EM, et al. Hypothermia during cardiopulmonary bypass increases need for inotropic support but does not impact inflammation in children undergoing surgical ventricular septal defect closure. Artificial Organs. 2016;**40**(5):470-479. DOI: 10.1111/aor.12587

[89] Stocker CF, Shekerdemian LS, Horton SB, Lee KJ, Eyres R, D'Udekem Y, et al. The influence of bypass temperature on the systemic

inflammatory response and organ injury after pediatric open surgery: A randomized trial. The Journal of Thoracic and Cardiovascular Surgery. 2011;**142**(1):174-180. DOI: 10.1016/j.jtcvs

[90] Staveski SL, Boulanger K, Erman L. The impact of massage and reading on children's pain and anxiety after cardiovascular surgery: A pilot study. Pediatric Critical Care Medicine. 2018;**19**(8):725-732. DOI: 10.1097/PCC.0000000000001615